MILADY'S STANDARD
THEORY
WORKBOOK
REVISED

MILADY'S STANDARD
THEORY
WORKBOOK
REVISED

To be used with
MILADY'S STANDARD TEXTBOOK OF COSMETOLOGY

Compiled by Linnea Lindquist,
Minneapolis Technical College

MILADY PUBLISHING COMPANY
(A Division of Delmar Publishers Inc.)
3 Columbia Circle, Box 12519
Albany, New York 12212-2519

Delmar Publishers' Online Services

To access Delmar on the World Wide Web, point your browser to:

http://www.delmar.com/delmar.html

To access through Gopher: gopher://gopher.delmar.com

(Delmar Online is part of "thomson.com", an Internet site with information on
more than 30 publishers of the International Thomson Publishing organization.)

For information on our products and services:

email: info@delmar.com

or call 800-347-7707

Revision Editor: Barbara Jewett

Photographer: Gillette Research Institue

Artists: Edward Tadiello
Judy Francis
Shizuko Horii
Cynthia Saniewski
CEM
Nelva Richardson

For information address:
Milady Publishing Company
(A Division of Delmar Publishers Inc.)
3 Columbia Circle, Box 12519
Albany, NY 12212-2519

Printed in the United States of America
Printed and published simultaneously in Canada

9 10 XXX 01 00 99 98 97

Library of Congress Catalog Card Number: 93–26375

ISBN: 1–56253–220–0

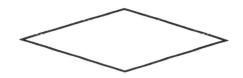

Contents

How to Use This Workbook

Milady's Standard Theory Workbook has been written to meet the needs, interests, and abilities of students receiving training in cosmetology.

This workbook should be used together with *Milady's Standard Textbook of Cosmetology (Revised)* and *Milady's Standard Practical Workbook.* This book directly follows the theoretical information found in the student textbook. Pages to be read and studied are listed at the beginning of each chapter. The practical information can be found in *Milady's Standard Practical Workbook.*

Students are to answer each item in this workbook with a pencil after consulting their textbook for correct information. Items can be corrected and/or rated during class or individual discussions, or on an independent study basis.

Various tests are included to emphasize essential facts found in the textbook and to measure the student's progress. "Word Reviews" are listed for each chapter. They are to be used as study guides, for class discussions, or for the teacher to assign groups of words to be used by the student in creative essays.

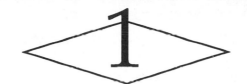

Date _____
Rating _____
Text Pages 9–22

YOUR PROFESSIONAL IMAGE

PERSONAL AND PROFESSIONAL HEALTH

1. Name eight guidelines for maintaining a healthy body and mind.

   1. _____ 2. _____

   3. _____ 4. _____

   5. _____ 6. _____

   7. _____ 8. _____

2. What four items are affected by what you eat?

   1. _____ 2. _____

   3. _____ 4. _____

3. Define personal hygiene. _____

4. Personal cleanliness aids in the maintenance of good health. Check off the practices that contribute to personal cleanliness.

   _____ daily bath or shower

   _____ daily use of deodorant

   _____ daily cleansing of teeth

   _____ monthly cleansing of face

   _____ daily grooming and cleansing of hair

   _____ the common use of towels

   _____ daily grooming and cleansing of nails

5. Outline the requirements for proper foot care.

   1. _____

   2. _____

   3. _____

   4. _____

   5. _____

   6. _____

1

PHYSICAL PRESENTATION

6. What are the three parts of your physical presentation?

   1. _____ 2. _____

   3. _____

7. Identify the defective body posture shown in the illustration below.

1. _____ 2. _____ 3. _____ 4. _____ 5. _____

   _____   _____   _____   _____   _____

8. List four items that a good physical presentation prevents.

   1. _____ 2. _____

   3. _____ 4. _____

9. Give five rules for a proper sitting position.

   1. _____

   2. _____

   3. _____

   4. _____

   5. _____

PERSONALITY

10. Define personality.

   _____

11. Name the ways in which you express your personality.

1. _____   2. _____
3. _____   4. _____
5. _____   6. _____
7. _____   8. _____
9. _____   10. _____

12. List five ways in which you may show good manners to other people.

1. _____
2. _____
3. _____
4. _____
5. _____

COMMUNICATION

13. Communication includes the following five items:

1. _____   2. _____
3. _____   4. _____
5. _____

HUMAN RELATIONS AND YOUR PROFESSIONAL ATTITUDE

14. Define human relations. _____

15. When talking with your client, it may be best to avoid discussing controversial topics. Controversial topics include:

1. _____   2. _____
3. _____   4. _____
5. _____   6. _____

TO BE SUCCESSFUL

16. List five things that will help you to be successful.

1. _____   2. _____
3. _____   4. _____
5. _____

PROFESSIONAL ETHICS

17. Define ethics. _____

18. Ethics is also a code of _____ by which you conduct yourself.

19. Write down two rules of ethics that students should practice.

1. _____

2. _____

20. Unethical practices affect the:

1. _____ 2. _____

3. _____ 4. _____

WORD REVIEW

appearance	exercise	neat
attitude	fatigue	nutrition
behavior	grooming	personality
clean	habits	podiatrist
communication	health	polite
conduct	honesty	posture
confidence	human relations	professional
conversation	humor	public
cosmetology	hygiene	relaxation
courtesy	mannerisms	respect
deodorant	manners	rest
diet	massage	successful
ethics	muscle	

BACTERIOLOGY

1. Bacteriology is the science that deals with the study of microorganisms called

    _____

2. As a cosmetologist, you must understand how the spread of disease can be prevented in order to protect the health of:

    1. _____   2. _____

3. Contagious diseases are caused by:

    1. _____

    2. _____

    3. _____

4. Define bacteria.

    _____

5. Bacteria are also known as: _____ or _____.

6. List seven places where bacteria may exist.

    1. _____   2. _____

    3. _____   4. _____

    5. _____   6. _____

    7. _____

7. With which instrument can bacteria be seen? _____

8. Name the two types of bacteria.

    1. _____   2. _____

9. The type of bacteria that is helpful or harmless is _____.

10. The type of bacteria that is harmful is _____.

11. Three types of pathogenic bacteria are:

    1. _____   2. _____

    3. _____

12. Identify the various forms of bacteria illustrated below.

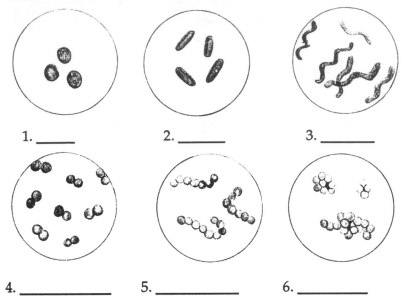

1. _____   2. _____   3. _____

4. _____   5. _____   6. _____

13. Matching: *Match the terms on the left with their correct descriptions on the right.*

____ 1. spirilla   A.   cause boils

____ 2. streptococci   B.   cause pneumonia

____ 3. diplococci   C.   round-shaped bacteria

____ 4. flagella   D.   cell division

____ 5. cocci   E.   active stage

____ 6. spherical spores   F.   rod-shaped bacteria

____ 7. staphylococci   G.   nonpathogenic bacteria

____ 8. mitosis   H.   curved or corkscrew-shaped bacteria

____ 9. bacilli   I.   hairlike projections for movement

                                    J.   cause strep throat

                                    K.   tough outer covering

                                    L.   diamond-shaped bacteria

14. Name the two phases in the bacterial life cycle.

    1. _____   2. _____

15. Bacteria grow and multiply best when the environment is:

    1. _____   2. _____

    3. _____   4. _____

16. What happens to bacteria when conditions are unfavorable?

    _____

17. What happens to inactive bacterial spores when favorable conditions are restored?

    _____

18. When does an infection occur?

    _____

19. Name two kinds of infections.

    1. _____   2. _____

20. Syphilis is an example of a _____ infection.

21. A boil or a pimple is an example of a _____ infection.

22. Define contagious or communicable.

_____

23. List six of the more common contagious diseases that prevent cosmetologists from working.

    1. _____   2. _____

    3. _____   4. _____

    5. _____   6. _____

24. Name the four ways pathogenic bacteria can enter the body.

    1. _____   2. _____

    3. _____   4. _____

25. What are the four ways the body fights infection?

    1. _____   2. _____

    3. _____   4. _____

26. Name two body secretions that discourage bacterial growth.

    1. _____   2. _____

27. What should the cosmetologist do with clients who have infectious diseases?

_____

28. Matching: *Match the terms on the left with their correct descriptions on the right.*

    ___ 1. parasites   A.   destroys all bacteria

    ___ 2. animal parasites   B.   molds, mildews, and yeasts

    ___ 3. filterable viruses   C.   developed by the body after overcoming a

    ___ 4. acquired immunity   disease

    ___ 5. plant parasites   D.   natural resistance to disease

    ___ 6. natural immunity   E.   cause the common cold

                              F.   vegetable bacterial stage

                              G.   organisms that live on other living organisms

                              H.   spore-forming bacterial stage

                              I.   itch mites and head lice

29. Acquired Immune Deficiency Syndrome is also known as _____ and is caused by the _____ virus.

30. AIDS may lie dormant in an infected person's system for up to _____ years.

31. Name three ways HIV *cannot* be transferred.

    1. _____   2. _____

    3. _____

32. List four ways the AIDS virus can be transferred.

    1. _____

    2. _____

    3. _____

    4. _____

33. How can AIDS be transferred in the salon? _____

WORD REVIEW

Acquired Immune Deficiency Syndrome	germ	protoplasm
active	head lice	reproduction
bacilli	immunity	ringworm
bacteria	inactive	saprophytes
bacteriology	infection	scabies
cilia	inoculation	spherical spores
cocci	microbe	spirilla
communicable	microorganisms	spore
contagious	microscope	staphylococci
daughter cells	mitosis	streptococci
diphtheria	motility	syphilis
diplococci	nonpathogenic	tetanus
filterable	parasite	typhoid
flagella	pathogenic	vegetative
	pediculosis	virus

DECONTAMINATION AND INFECTION CONTROL

INTRODUCTION

1. A clean salon promotes clients' confidence in _____.

2. Protecting against the spread of infectious germs and organisms is required by

   _____.

3. Careless actions cause _____ and _____.

PREVENTION AND CONTROL

4. Removing pathogens and other substances from tools or surfaces is called

   _____.

5. List the three main levels of decontamination.

   1. _____   2. _____

   3. _____

6. Which of the above are useful in the salon? _____

7. Define sterilization. _____

8. Name two physical methods of sterilization.

   1. _____   2. _____

9. Name two occupations that must practice sterilization.

   1. _____   2 _____

10. Sterilization is an _____ decontamination method for salons.

11. Define sanitation. _____

12. How are salon tools and other surfaces sanitized?

    _____

13. Sanitized surfaces may still harbor _____.

14. List three examples of sanitation.

    1. _____

    2. _____

    3. _____

15. Which government agency oversees salon sanitation?

_____

16. A solution that is safe to use on skin is an _____ .

17. Define disinfection.

_____

_____

18. Substances that kill microbes on contaminated tools and other nonliving surfaces are called

_____ .

19. Where should disinfectants not be used? _____

20. Safe use of disinfectants requires using _____

21. All disinfectants must be approved for use by the

_____ .

22. To prevent accidental exposure, wear _____ and _____ when working with disinfectants.

23. What does OSHA stand for? _____

24. List four types of information that should be present on a Material Safety Data Sheet.

   1. _____   2. _____

   3. _____   4. _____

25. Identify two functions of a hospital level disinfectant.

   1. _____   2. _____

26. Before soaking in a disinfecting solution, all implements should be thoroughly _____ .

27. Jars or containers used to disinfect implements are called _____ .

28. To avoid spreading pathogens, never touch a client's _____ and be sure

   to _____ any implement that comes in contact.

TYPES OF DISINFECTANTS

29. Identification Match: *Using the letters Q, PH, SH, and A (as defined below), match the characteristics listed below with the correct disinfectant.*

    Key:

    Q=quaternary ammonium compounds, or quats
    PH=phenols
    SH=sodium hypochlorite
    A=alcohol

    Characteristics:

    _____   1. safe and fast acting

    _____   2. flammable

    _____   3. also known as common household bleach

    _____   4. disinfects implements in 10 to 15 minutes

    _____   5. 99% isopropyl equals the strength of 70% ethyl

    _____   6. may soften or discolor rubber and plastic

    _____   7. effective for cleaning tables and counter tops

    _____   8. can seriously burn skin and eyes

    _____   9. can corrode tools and dull sharp edges

    _____   10. may be poisonous if accidentally ingested

30. Describe how an ultrasonic bath works.

    _____

    _____

31. How should disinfectants be stored? _____

32. What disinfectant is no longer considered safe for salon use? _____

33. What type of hand soap should a salon use? _____

34. List the six steps to properly disinfect a surface.

    1. _____   2. _____

    3. _____   4. _____

    5. _____   6. _____

35. Name three ways to properly store disinfected tools.

    1. _____   2. _____

    3. _____

UNIVERSAL SANITATION

36. Name four things that must be done to protect yourself and your clients.

    1. _____   2. _____

    3. _____   4. _____

WORD REVIEW

alcohol	disinfectant	sanitation
antiseptic	EPA	sodium hypochlorite
bactericide	fungicide	sterilization
contagious	MSDS	ultrasonic cleaner
contaminant	OSHA	universal sanitation
contaminated	phenols	virucide
decontamination	quats	wet sanitizer

Date _____
Rating _____
Text Pages 43-66

PROPERTIES OF THE SCALP AND HAIR

HAIR

1. The study of hair is called _____.

2. The two main purposes of hair are:

    1. _____   2. _____

3. Hair is an appendage of the _____.

4. The name of the protein that hair is made of is _____.

5. Average hair is composed of:

    1. _____% carbon   2. _____% hydrogen

    3. _____% nitrogen   4. _____% sulfur

    5. _____% oxygen

6. The hair root is located _____ the skin surface. It has three main structures:

    1. _____   2. _____

    3. _____

7. Identify the parts of the skin and hair illustrated below.

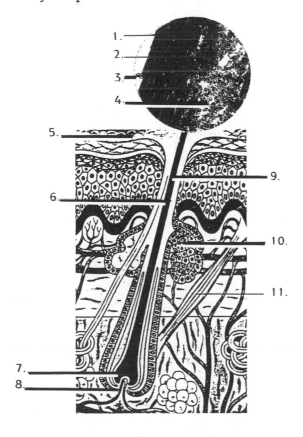

1. _____

2. _____

3. _____

4. _____

5. _____

6. _____

7. _____

8. _____

9. _____

10. _____

_____

11. _____

13

8. Within the hair papilla is a rich blood and nerve supply that contributes to the

   _____ and _____ of the hair.

9. Straight hair is usually _____ in shape. Wavy hair is usually _____ in shape.

   Curly, kinky hair is almost _____ in shape.

10. The _____ of a hair as it projects out of the follicle determines each person's hair shape.

11. Matching: *Match the terms on the left with their correct descriptions on the right.*

    ____ 1. follicle   A.   club-shaped structure in the lower root

    ____ 2. arrector pili   B.   hair flowing in the same direction

    ____ 3. sebum   C.   a tuft of hair that stays down

    ____ 4. whorl   D.   involuntary muscle

    ____ 5. bulb   E.   hair that forms a circular pattern

    ____ 6. cowlick   F.   tubelike depression that encases the hair root

    ____ 7. hair stream   G.   the first 1" of hair

    ____ 8. papilla   H.   oil that gives luster and pliability

    ____ 9. sebaceous gland   I.   cone-shaped elevation located at the bottom of the follicle

                              J.   ability of hair to absorb

                              K.   a tuft of hair standing up

                              L.   oil gland

12. The outside layer of the hair is the _____. The cells, which point away from the scalp, have the following three characteristics:

    1. _____   2. _____

    3. _____

13. The middle layer of the hair is the _____, which gives hair its strength and

    _____. This layer contains the _____ that gives the hair its color.

14. The innermost layer of hair is the _____ and is composed of cells that are

    _____ in shape.

15. List the three types of hair on the body.

    1. _____   2. _____

    3. _____

16. Hair on the face is called _____.

    Hair on the head is called _____.

    Hair of the eyelashes is called _____.

    Hair of the eyebrows is called _____.

17. The three cycles of hair growth are:

    1. _____   2. _____

    3. _____

18. On average, hair grows _____ inch per month.

19. How do climates and/or seasons affect hair?

    1. _____

    2. _____

    3. _____

20. Average daily shedding is between _____ and _____ hairs.

21. If the papilla is destroyed, will hair continue to grow? _____

22. What is the average life of hair? _____

23. Write down the amounts of hair per head according to hair color.

    1. blonde: _____   2. brown: _____

    3. black: _____   4. red: _____

24. Explain in four steps the sequence of natural replacement of hair.

    1. _____

    2. _____

    3. _____

    4. _____

    _____

25. The hair's coloring matter, called _____, is found in the hair's _____ layer.

26. Gray hair is caused by the _____ of color pigment.

HAIR ANALYSIS

27. List four senses you use in determining hair condition.

    1. _____   2. _____

    3. _____   4. _____

28. Define hair texture.

    _____

29. Variations in texture are due to:

    1. _____   2. _____

30. What type of finish does wiry hair have? _____

31. Define hair porosity. _____

32. List four types of porosity.

    1. _____   2. _____

    3. _____   4. _____

33. Define elasticity.

    _____

34. List three classifications of elasticity.

   1. _____   2. _____

   3. _____

35. Wet hair can be stretched _____% to _____% of its length.

36. Matching: *Match the terms on the left with their correct descriptions on the right.*

   ___ 1. congenital canities   A.   alternate bands of gray and dark hair

   ___ 2. acquired canities   B.   split hair ends

   ___ 3. ringed hair   C.   moist hair

   ___ 4. hypertrichosis   D.   gray hair at birth

   ___ 5. trichoptilosis   E.   very curly hair

   ___ 6. trichorrhexis nodosa   F.   knotted hair

   ___ 7. monilethrix   G.   brittle hair

   ___ 8. fragilitas crinium   H.   superfluous hair

                                     I.   very straight hair

                                     J.   gray hair due to old age

                                     K.   beaded hair

Also see *Milady's Standard Practical Workbook.*

WORD REVIEW

acquired canities	fine	oxygen
adornment	follicle	papilla
albino	fragilitas crinium	pigment
appendage	gray	porosity
arrector pili	growth	protection
barba	hair cycle	protein
bulb	hair root	replacement
canities	hair shaft	sebaceous gland
capilia	hair stream	sebum
carbon	hydrogen	sulfur
cilia	hypertrichosis	supercilia
coarse	keratin	superfluous
congenital canities	lanugo	texture
cortex	medium	trichology
cowlick	medulla	trichoptilosis
cuticle	melanin	trichorrhexis nodosa
density	monilethrix	whorl
elasticity	nitrogen	wiry
fall		

DRAPING

See *Milady's Standard Practical Workbook.*

SHAMPOOING, RINSING, AND CONDITIONING

TYPES OF SHAMPOOS

1. The highest dollar expenditure in hair care products is for (check one):

    _____ home permanents

    _____ shampoo

2. It is the cosmetologist's responsibility to understand the _____ composition of a shampoo

    in order to _____ the best type for a client.

3. The letters pH stand for: _____ .

4. What is the range of a pH scale? _____

5. The amount of _____ in a solution determines whether it is more alkaline or more

    _____ .

6. The higher the pH, the stronger and _____ the shampoo, which can leave the hair dry and _____ .

7. Identification Match: *Using the letters A, C, M, and D (as defined below), match the correct characteristics listed below with one of the types of shampoos.*

    Key:

    A=acid-balanced shampoo
    C=conditioning shampoo
    M=medicated shampoo
    D=powder dry shampoo

    Characteristics:

    _____ 1. contains agents that make hair smooth and shiny

    _____ 2. additives may be citric, lactic, or phosphoric

    _____ 3. reduces excess dandruff

    _____ 4. contains special drugs

    _____ 5. falls within 4.5–6.6 pH range

    _____ 6. given when a client's health does not permit a wet shampoo

    _____ 7. improves manageability of hair

    _____ 8. prescribed by a physician

    _____ 9. not to be used before a chemical service

HAIR RINSES

8. What four items are mixed together to make a hair rinse?

1. _____

2. _____

3. _____

4. _____

9. Identification Match: *Using the letters AR, CC, AB, MR, and CL (as defined below), match the correct characteristics listed below with one type of rinse.*

Key:

AR=acid rinse
CC=conditioner and cream rinse
AB=acid-balanced rinse
MR=medicated rinse
CL=color rinse

Characteristics:

_____ 1. intended to soften and untangle hair

_____ 2. adds temporary color to the hair

_____ 3. removes soap scum from the hair

_____ 4. prevents fading of color

_____ 5. controls minor dandruff problems

_____ 6. restores the pH balance

_____ 7. closes the cuticle to trap in color molecules

_____ 8. temporarily coats the hair

_____ 9. citric, tartaric, acetic, and lactic

_____ 10. habitual use can lead to a build up

_____ 11. remains on the hair until the next shampoo

Also see *Milady's Standard Practical Workbook.*

WORD REVIEW

acetic acid	color rinse	pH
acid	conditioner	pH scale
acid-balanced rinse	conditioning shampoo	phosphoric acid
acid-balanced shampoo	cream rinse	potential hydrogen
acid rinse	lactic acid	powder dry shampoo
alkaline	medicated rinse	shampoo
citric acid	medicated shampoo	tartaric acid
color/highlighting shampoo		

HAIRCUTTING

See *Milady's Standard Practical Workbook.*

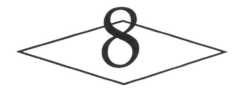

FINGER WAVING

See *Milady's Standard Practical Workbook.*

WET HAIRSTYLING

See *Milady's Standard Practical Workbook.*

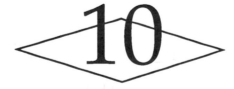

THERMAL HAIRSTYLING

See *Milady's Standard Practical Workbook.*

Date _____
Rating _____
Text Pages 187–224

PERMANENT WAVING

INTRODUCTION

1. List four benefits that perming gives to both the client and stylist.

   1. _____

   2. _____

   3. _____

   4. _____

HISTORY OF PERMANENT WAVING

2. In 1905, a wired machine that supplied _____ was invented by Charles Nessler.

3. Winding hair from scalp to ends is a technique called _____.

4. Winding hair from ends to scalp is a technique called _____.

5. In 1931, the _____ perm method was introduced. This used _____ that were pre-heated.

6. The first _____ perm was developed in 1932. It used chemical pads that were

   _____ with water.

7. In 1941, a waving _____ was developed. It is a liquid that causes the hair to soften

   and _____.

8. A second lotion, which hardens and _____ the hair, is called a _____.

   It also stops the action of the _____ lotion.

9. Why is a cold wave called a "cold wave?" _____

10. Two perming terms/words that are used synonymously are:

   1. _____   2. _____

11. Introduced in 1970, perms with a pH range of 4.5 to 7.9 are called _____

   _____ perms.

12. Neutral and acid-balanced perms require that the client be placed under a heated dryer. What are two reasons for this?

   1. _____   2. _____

MODERN PERM CHEMISTRY

13. To ensure optimum curl development, stop action _____ is incorporated into many waving _____ .

14. List the two chemical steps in the perming process.

    1. _____   2. _____

15. What is the main active ingredient in alkaline perms? _____

16. This (number 15 above) ingredient is a compound made up of _____ and

    _____ .

17. Generally speaking, alkaline perms have a pH range of _____, depending on the amount of the ingredient _____ in them.

18. What does an alkaline do to the cuticle layer? _____

19. Whose directions do you follow when giving a perm? _____

20. List three benefits of alkaline perms.

    1. _____   2. _____

    3. _____

21. When should you use an alkaline perm?

    1. _____

    2. _____

    3. _____

22. The main ingredient in acid-balanced waving lotions is glyceryl _____, which gives these perms a pH range of _____ .

23. What are the two ways heat is used in acid-balanced perms?

    1. _____

    2. _____

24. List three benefits of acid-balanced perms.

    1. _____

    2. _____

    3. _____

25. When should acid-balanced perms be used?

    1. _____

    2. _____

    3. _____

26. What permanently establishes the new curl shape? _____

27. What may happen if the hair is not properly neutralized?

_____

28. What is the name of the oxidizing agent that is in neutralizers? _____

29. List two reasons why you should carefully read and follow the directions for each perm.

   1. _____   2. _____

HAIR STRUCTURE AND PERMING

30. Name the two actions of all perms.

   1. _____

   2. _____

31. Which layer of the hair must open to allow the chemicals to enter? _____

32. In which layer of the hair do the physical and chemical actions take place? _____

33. Which layer of the hair is probably not affected by a perm? _____

34. Keratin is made up of 19 _____ acids. These bond together to form a

   _____ chain.

35. Cysteine is joined together with _____ bonds, which must be broken down to allow
   for perming.

36. List the two actions that the waving lotion does to the hair.

   1. _____   2. _____

37. What two actions does the neutralizer do to the hair?

   1. _____   2. _____

Also see *Milady's Standard Practical Workbook*.

WORD REVIEW

acid-balanced perm	endothermic	permanent waving
alkaline perm	exothermic	perming
amino acids	glyceryl monothioglycolate	physical action
ammonia	hardens and shrinks	polypeptide chain
ammonium thioglycolate	hydrogen peroxide	pre-heat perm
blocking	keratin	processing
chemical action	machine perm	reducing agent
client consultation	machineless perm	sectioning
cold waves	manual dexterity	softens and expands
cortex	manufacturer's directions	spiral wrapping
croquignole wrapping	medulla	stop action processing
cuticle	Nessler (Charles)	thioglycolic acid
cysteine	neutralizer	waving lotion
disulfide bonds	oxidizing agent	wrapping

HAIRCOLORING

INTRODUCTION

1. List four processes of haircoloring.

   1. _adding artificial pigment to the natural haircolor_
   2. _adding artificial pigment to previously colored hair_
   3. _ "   "   "   to prelightened hair._
   4. _diffusing natural pigment & adding artificial pigment in one step._

2. List four processes for decolorizing, or lightening, the hair.

   1. _decolorizing to prepare for final color_ 2. _decolorizing the natural or artificial pigment to desired color._
   3. _corrective color_ 4. _selected areas highlighting._

3. Why do people color or lighten their hair?

   1. _graying_ 2. _Self-Image Boost_
   3. _experimental_ 4. _artistic_
   5. _corrective_

CONSULTATION AND ANALYSIS

4. Name the five communication steps important for a good client consultation.

   1. _greeting_
   2. _appearance_ → _use of professional industry terminology_
   3. _credibility_
   4. _personal appearance_
   5. _confident mannerisms_

5. State why hair structure is important. _Because products cause a dramatic change_

6. When a product significantly changes the hair structure, the resulting hair strand is _weaker_.

7. Every hair on a person's head is composed of these three parts: _the cuticle cortex and medulla_

8. The diameter of the individual hair strand is called the _hair texture_.

9. The terms coarse, medium, and fine are used to differentiate between _large, medium and small diameter_

10. Define porosity. _ability of hair to absob moisture_

11. Describe hair density. _number of hairs per square inch on the scalp._

12. List the three types of hair formation.

    1. _Straight_   2. _wavy_

    3. _Curly_

IDENTIFYING THE NATURAL HAIR COLOR

13. Natural pigments are classified as _melanins_, which are made of molecules capable of

    reflecting _color_.

14. Eumelanin is classified as _blk-brown_ and pheomelanin is classified as _yellow-red_

15. The natural hair color tone we see is determined by the _melanin -eumelanin, pheomelanin, or a combination of both_

    present. The lightness or darkness of the tone is determined by the _amount and distribution_ of the melanin.

16. The degree of lightness or darkness of a particular color, excluding tone, is called the color

    _____.

17. Level systems colors are classified on a scale of 1 to 10, with 1 being _____ and 10

    being _____.

18. Explain how cosmetologists can identify the level and base color of the client's hair.

    _____

19. Define tone. _____

20. List the colors considered to be warm tones. _____

21. List the colors considered to be cool tones. _____

22. What are two other terms used for cool colors?

    1. _____   2. _____

23. Describe intensity. _____

COLOR THEORY

24. The Law of Color regulates the mixing of dyes and pigment to make other _____.

25. List the three primary colors.

    1. _____   2. _____

    3. _____

26. The easiest primary color to remove from the hair shaft is _____.

27. Describe how to remove red color from the hair shaft.

    _____

    _____

28. Complete removal of yellow from the hair shaft is best accomplished by _____.

29. Adding yellow to your color mixture will make a color appear _____.

30. When all three primary colors are present in equal proportions, the resulting color is _____.

31. List the three secondary colors.

    1. _____   2. _____

    3. _____

32. How do we create secondary colors?

_____

33. List six tertiary colors.

    1. _____   2. _____

    3. _____   4. _____

    5. _____   6. _____

34. How do we create tertiary colors?

_____

35. Draw a color wheel and place the primary, secondary, and tertiary colors on it in their proper places.

36. What are complementary colors?

_____

37. When mixed together, complementary colors _____ each other.

38. To neutralize unwanted orange ("brassy") tone, use a haircolor product with a _____ base.

39. To neutralize unwanted yellow tone, use a haircolor product with yellow's complementary

color of _____.

CLASSIFICATIONS OF HAIRCOLORING

40. Name four categories of haircolor.

    1. _____   2. _____

    3. _____   4. _____

41. Temporary colors last from _____ to _____ because the color

_____.

42. Identify two situations where temporary colors are valuable.

1. _____

2. _____

43. List the types of temporary colors.

1. _____   2. _____

3. _____   4. _____

5. _____   6. _____

7. _____

44. Semi-permanent colors last four to _____ shampoos, and gently deposit color in the

cortex layer, as well as coat the hair's _____ layer.

45. Deposit-only haircolors use _____ to gently swell and open the

cuticle layer and drive the color into the _____.

46. Deposit-only colors last four to six _____, gradually fading from the hair and

producing a diffused line of _____.

47. List five situations where deposit-only color is a good choice.

1. _____

2. _____

3. _____

4. _____

5. _____

48. Deposit-only color will _____ the natural hair color when applied, so select a shade

_____ than the client's natural shade.

49. Permanent color penetrates the cuticle layer and _____ molecules into the hair's

_____ layer. This type of haircolor product can both lift and _____ color into
the hair.

50. What needs to be done if a permanent color contains aniline derivatives?

_____

51. Identification Match: *Using the letters OX, VT, MD, and CD (as defined below), match the correct characteristics listed below with one type of haircoloring.*

    Key:

    OX=oxidation tints
    VT=vegetable tints
    MD=metallic dyes
    CD=compound dyes

    Characteristics:

    _____ 1. has a coating action that can build up

    _____ 2. can lighten and deposit color in one process

    _____ 3. ingredients react with keratin and turn the hair brown

    _____ 4. advertised as "color restorers" or "progressive colors"

    _____ 5. also known as an aniline derivative, penetrating, synthetic-organic, and amino tints

    _____ 6. metallic salts are added for their staying power

    _____ 7. made from herbs, flowers, and plants

    _____ 8. combines metallic dyes with vegetable tints

    _____ 9. are mixed with hydrogen peroxide

    _____ 10. henna is still used today

52. Metals in dyes will fade to some very unnatural tones. Silver dyes can have a _____ cast, lead can have a _____ cast, and copper may turn the color _____.

53. What two products do you mix together in order to test hair for metallic salts and dyes?

    1. _____ 2. _____

54. If this mixture (item number 53 above) causes the hair to boil, it tells you that _____ is present. If it lightens immediately, it tells you that _____ is present.

55. The best way to guarantee that these metals are removed from the hair is to _____ the hair.

HYDROGEN PEROXIDE

56. The oxidizing agent most commonly used in haircoloring is _____. It is distributed under a variety of names, such as the following four terms:

    1. _____ 2. _____

    3. _____ 4. _____

57. The three forms of hydrogen peroxide are:

    1. _____ 2. _____

    3. _____

58. Which form can boost the volume? _____

59. What is added to cream peroxide for control? _____

60. 3.5 to 4.0 is the pH of which type of peroxide? _____

61. Most coloring products use _____ volume hydrogen peroxide, although using 40 volume will result in a _____ color. Using lower than 20 volume will allow more _____ than lift.

62. What device is used to measure the volume of liquid hydrogen peroxide? _____

63. Do not allow hydrogen peroxide formulations to come in contact with any _____.

HAIR LIGHTENING

64. Define hair lightening. _____

65. Briefly list the two purposes of lighteners.

    1. _____

    2. _____

66. What four things must you consider in order to achieve the desired shade?

    1. _____

    2. _____

    3. _____

    4. _____

67. List seven actions of hair lighteners.

    1. _____

    2. _____

    3. _____

    4. _____

    5. _____

    6. _____

    7. _____

68. List three types of lighteners.

    1. _____   2. _____

    3. _____

69. What are four benefits of cream lighteners?

    1. _____

    2. _____

    3. _____

    4. _____

70. Powder lighteners are too harsh to use close to the scalp, and so they are generally used for _____ lightening.

71. List the ten stages of lightening.

1. _____   2. _____

3. _____   4. _____

5. _____   6. _____

7. _____   8. _____

9. _____   10. _____

GRAY HAIR CHALLENGES AND SOLUTIONS

72. Describe gray hair. _____

73. Define salt-and-pepper hair.

_____

74. Both gray and white hair contain little _____ within the _____ .

75. List four causes of yellowed gray hair.

1. _____   2. _____

3. _____   4. _____

76. Yellow discoloration occurring from internal causes or the oxidation of melanin can be

removed with _____ .

77. Name two other methods of treating yellowed gray hair.

1. _____

2. _____

Also see *Milady's Standard Practical Workbook.*

WORD REVIEW

amino tints	hydrogen peroxide	primary colors
aniline derivative tints	hydrometer	quaternary colors
certified colors	Law of Color	saturation
complementary colors	level	secondary colors
compound dyes	liquid lighteners	semi-permanent colors
cool colors	liquid peroxide	seven stages of lightening
cream lighteners	metallic/mineral dyes	synthetic-organic tints
cream peroxide	neutralize	temporary colors
deposit-only colors	oxidation tints	tertiary colors
diffusing	patch test	tint
drabbers	penetrating tints	tone
dry peroxide	permanent colors	toner
FDA	pigment	vegetable tints
haircoloring	powder lightener	volume
hair lightening	predisposition test	warm colors

CHEMICAL HAIR RELAXING AND SOFT CURL PERMANENT

INTRODUCTION

1. Define chemical hair relaxing.

   _____

   _____

CHEMICAL HAIR RELAXING PRODUCTS

2. List the three basic relaxing products.

   1. _____   2. _____

   3. _____

3. The two general types of relaxers are:

   1. _____   2. _____

4. Which of the two types of relaxers does NOT require pre-shampooing? _____

5. The solution enters the hair's _____ layer, where it breaks the sulfur and

   _____ bonds.

6. List the three items that act to smooth the hair.

   1. _____   2. _____

   3. _____

7. What is the pH factor of a sodium hydroxide relaxer? _____

8. Name the two actions that can happen if a lot of sodium hydroxide with a very high pH is used on a client.

   1. _____

   2. _____

9. What is less drastic in its action than sodium hydroxide? _____

10. This (number 9 above) chemical used in relaxing is the same solution that is used in

    _____.

11. Two other terms for neutralizer are:

    1. _____   2. _____

12. What does the neutralizer do to the hair?

    _____

13. A thio neutralizer reforms the _____ cross-bonds.

14. Name the two formulas of sodium hydroxide relaxers.

    1. _____ 2. _____

15. A petroleum cream is found in which type of relaxer? _____

16. This petroleum cream protects:

    1. _____ 2. _____

17. At body temperature, petroleum cream _____ to assure complete coverage of the

    client's _____. It also helps to prevent burning and/or _____ of the skin and
    scalp.

18. Name two distinct characteristics of a no-base relaxer.

    1. _____ 2. _____

STEPS IN CHEMICAL HAIR RELAXING

19. The three basic steps in relaxing are:

    1. _____ 2. _____

    3. _____

20. In which step does the hair begin to soften? _____

21. In what form does a neutralizer often come? _____

22. The conditioner in a relaxer may be applied before or _____ the relaxing treatment.

    This is determined by the _____.

23. The strength of relaxer to be used is determined by the _____ test.

24. List three relaxer strengths.

    1. _____ 2. _____

    3. _____

CHEMICAL HAIR RELAXING PROCESS

25. What is a different chemical, besides sodium hydroxide, that is used to relax the hair?

    _____

26. Is a thio relaxer stronger or weaker than a sodium hydroxide relaxer? _____

27. If using a thio relaxer, when is the hair shampooed? _____

28. If using a sodium hydroxide relaxer, when is the hair shampooed?

    _____

Also see *Milady's Standard Practical Workbook.*

WORD REVIEW

alkaline
ammonium thioglycolate
base formula
chemical hair relaxing
conditioning
cortical layer
cross-bonds
cysteine cross-bonds
fixative
hair straightener

hydrogen bonds
mild strength
neutralizer
neutralizing
no-base formula
overly curly hair
petroleum cream
pH
pre-shampooing

processing
protective base
regular strength
shampoo neutralizer
sodium hydroxide
stabilizer
strength of relaxers
strong/super strength
sulfur bonds

THERMAL HAIR STRAIGHTENING (HAIR PRESSING)

See *Milady's Standard Practical Workbook.*

THE ARTISTRY OF ARTIFICIAL HAIR

INTRODUCTION

1. The ancient Egyptians wore wigs to _____ .

2. List the three items related to wigs that can increase salon income.

   1. _____   2. _____

   3. _____

3. What four items must you learn in order to offer the best possible wig and hairpiece services?

   1. _____

   2. _____

   3. _____

   4. _____

WHY PEOPLE WEAR WIGS

4. List four reasons why people wear wigs.

   1. _____   2. _____

   3. _____   4. _____

5. Wigs are used by many people who have lost their natural hair. List three reasons why people experience hair loss.

   1. _____   2. _____

   3. _____

TYPES OF WIGS

6. List the four types of hair used in wigs.

   1. _____   2. _____

   3. _____   4. _____

7. To tell the difference between human and synthetic hair, take a lighted match and

   _____ a small piece of hair. If it gives off a strong odor, it is made of _____

   hair. If it gives off little or no odor, it is made of _____ hair.

8. Expensive wigs are _____ knotted into a mesh foundation. Cheaper wigs are sewn by

   _____ into a cap with rows.

9. List seven ways synthetic wigs and hairpieces closely resemble human hair.

    1. _____   2. _____

    3. _____   4. _____

    5. _____   6. _____

    7. _____

10. One characteristic of synthetic wigs is that of curl retention. Name three others.

    1. _____   2. _____

    3. _____

11. Which type of hair, synthetically produced or human, costs less? _____

12. In order to satisfy your client's needs of wear, comfort, and _____, you must consider

    quality, proper _____, and good _____ when selecting a wig.

13. An artificial hairpiece composed of rows of wefting sewn to elastic bands is called the

    _____. They are lighter and _____ than other types of wigs.

14. List six types of synthetic hairpieces.

    1. _____   2. _____

    3. _____   4. _____

    5. _____   6. _____

15. What type of hair is used to make extensions? _____

16. Name three purposes of extensions.

    1. _____   2. _____

    3. _____

17. How does a toupee stay on the head? _____

Also see *Milady's Standard Practical Workbook.*

WORD REVIEW

adhesive	hair replacements	nonflammable
animal hair	hairpieces	oxidize
braids	hand made	stretch wigs
cascades	human hair	synthetic
chignons	kanekalon	toupee
demi-wigs	machine made	venicelon
dynel	match test	weave
falls	modacrylic	wiglets
fitted wigs	no-cap wig	wigs
hair extensions		

Date _____
Rating _____
Text Pages 369–400

MANICURING AND PEDICURING

INTRODUCTION

1. What is the purpose of a manicure?

   _____

2. List six qualifications of a manicurist.

   1. _____
   2. _____
   3. _____
   4. _____
   5. _____

      _____
   6. _____

SHAPES OF NAILS

3. The four general nail shapes are:

   1. _____   2. _____
   3. _____   4. _____

4. For a more natural effect, the shape of the nail should conform to that of the _____.

5. Which nail shape fits most hands? _____

EQUIPMENT, IMPLEMENTS, COSMETICS, AND MATERIALS

6. List nine pieces of equipment needed in manicuring.

   1. _____
   2. _____
   3. _____
   4. _____
   5. _____
   6. _____
   7. _____
   8. _____
   9. _____

7. Matching: *Match the terms on the left with their correct descriptions on the right.*

____ 1. nail file   A.   shapes the free edge

____ 2. camel's hair brush   B.   trims and cuts the cuticle

____ 3. orangewood stick   C.   polishes and buffs the nail

____ 4. tweezers   D.   removes nail polish

____ 5. nail buffer   E.   wooden; for working around the nail

____ 6. cuticle pusher   F.   lifts small bits of cuticle

____ 7. cuticle nipper   G.   adds length to the nail

                                           H.   used to apply nail polish

                                           I.   reduces nail biting

                                           J.   used to loosen the cuticle

8. Dry nail polish smooths the nail and gives it a gloss during _____ (where permitted).

9. What can be used with a nail buffer to smooth nail ridges?

_____

10. Before applying colored polish to the nails, you are to apply a _____ coat. This allows the polish to _____ readily to the nail. It also prevents the color from _____ the nail tissue.

11. After applying colored polish to the nails, you are to apply a _____ coat. This protects the nail _____ and minimizes chipping or _____.

12. Matching: *Match the terms on the left with their correct descriptions on the right.*

____ 1. cuticle remover   A.   dissolves old polish on nails

____ 2. polish thinner   B.   acrylic nail applicator

____ 3. cuticle oil   C.   contains 2% to 5% sodium or potassium hydroxide

____ 4. hand creams   D.   removes stains on the nail

____ 5. nail whitener   E.   holds warm, soapy water

____ 6. alum   F.   softens and lubricates the skin around the nail

____ 7. nail polish   G.   protects nail polish against stickiness and dulling

____ 8. polish remover   H.   contains emollients, humectants, emulsifiers, and preservatives

____ 9. nail hardener   I.   keeps nail tips looking white

____ 10. cuticle cream   J.   used to rest client's arm

____ 11. nail dryer   K.   thins out thick nail polish

____ 12. nail bleach   L.   colors or glosses the nail

                                           M.   stops bleeding

                                           N.   lanolin, petroleum, or beeswax based

                                           O.   prevents nail from splitting or peeling

13. Briefly list twelve materials needed for manicuring.

1. _____   2. _____
3. _____   4. _____
5. _____   6. _____
7. _____   8. _____
9. _____   10. _____
11. _____   12. _____

Also see *Milady's Standard Practical Workbook.*

WORD REVIEW

abrasive
alum
antiseptic
base coat
cleanser
cura
cushion
cuticle cream
cuticle nippers
cuticle oil
cuticle pusher
cuticle remover
disinfectant
dry nail polish
electric heater
emery board
emollient
finger bowl

hand cream/lotion
humectants
lamp
liquid nail polish
manicure
manus
mending adhesive
mending tissue
nail bleach
nail brush
nail buffer
nail cleanser
nail dryer
nail file
nail hardener/
   strengthener
nail polish
nail polish thinner

nail technician
nail whitener
orangewood stick
oval shape
pointed shape
polish remover
pumice powder
round shape
70% alcohol
spatula
square shape
supply tray
table
top coat
towel
tweezers
wet sanitizer

Date _____
Rating _____
Text Pages 401–410

THE NAIL AND ITS DISORDERS

INTRODUCTION

1. The technical term for the nail is _____onyx_____.

2. The nail is an _____appendage_____ of the skin.

3. The color of a healthy nail is _____pink_____, and its surface is smooth, _____curved_____ and unspotted.

THE NAIL

4. The nail is made up mainly of a protein called _____Keratin_____. In appearance, the nail itself is whitish and _____pinkish_____. The nail plate contains no nerves or _____blood_____ vessels.

5. The three parts of the nail are the:
   1. _____nail body_____   2. _____nail root_____
   3. _____free edge_____

6. The visible portion of the nail is the nail _____body_____. It extends from the root to the _____free edge_____.

7. At the base of the nail is the nail _____root_____, which is attached to an actively growing tissue called the _____matrix_____.

8. The end portion that reaches over the fingertips is the _____free edge_____.

9. The skin on which the nail body rests is the nail _____bed_____. It has many _____blood_____ vessels and is abundantly supplied with _____nerves_____.

10. The matrix contains the following three items:
    1. _____nerves_____   2. _____lymph_____
    3. _____blood vessels_____

11. Three reasons why nail growth may be retarded are:
    1. _____poor health_____   2. _____nail disorder or disease_____
    3. _____injury to nail matrix_____.

12. The half-moon at the base of the nail is called the _____lunula_____.

13. Identify the parts of the nail illustrated below.

a.
1. _hyponychium_
2. _nail body_
3. _nail groove_
4. _nail bed_
5. _lunula_
6. _nail wall_
7. _nail matrix_
8. _nail root_

b.
1. _free edge_
2. _nail body_
3. _nail bed_
4. _eponychium_
5. _nail root_
6. _nail matrix_

STRUCTURES SURROUNDING THE NAIL

14. Matching: *Match the terms on the left with their correct descriptions on the right.*

_C_ 1. cuticle   A. extension of the cuticle at the base of the nail body
_J_ 2. nail walls   B. uneven nail growth
_H_ 3. mantle   C. overlapping skin around the nail
_D_ 4. nail grooves   D. slits along which the growing nail moves
_A_ 5. eponychium   E. white spots on the nail
_I_ 6. hyponychium   F. portion of the epidermis surrounding entire
_F_ 7. perionychium   nail border
                        G. half-moon at nail base
                        H. fold of skin with nail root embedded in it
                        I. portion of the epidermis under the free edge
                        J. folds of skin overlapping the nail sides

NAIL GROWTH

15. Three items that influence nail growth are:
    1. _nutrition_   2. _general health_
    3. _disease_

16. Nails, on an average, grow _1/8_ inch per month. They grow faster in the _summer_ season than in winter, and faster on _children_ than on the elderly. The one specific nail that grows the fastest is on the _middle_ finger.

17. If the nail bed is injured, the new nail growth will be _badly_ formed.

18. A nail will be replaced as long as the _matrix_ remains in good condition. Nail replacement takes about _four_ months.

NAIL DISORDERS

19. A nail technician should never treat nail _disease_. However, simple nail irregularities and _blemishes_ can be treated by the nail technician.

20. Briefly describe the following nail irregularities.

1. corrugations: *way ridges caused by uneven growth of nail*

2. furrows: *depression in the nails - usually the result of illness or injury to cells of nail matrix*

3. leuconychia: *white spots - caused by injury to base of nail*

4. onychauxis: *or hypertrophy — overgrowth of nail*

5. onychatrophia: *atrophy or wasting away of the nail*

6. pterygium: *is a forward growth of the cuticle that adheres to base of nail.*

7. onychophagy: _____

8. onychorrhexis: _____

9. hangnail/agnail: _____

10. eggshell nails: _____

11. blue nails: _____

12. bruised nail: _____

FUNGUS AND MOLD

21. _____ is the general term for vegetable parasites including all types of fungus and mold.

22. A discoloration in the nail that spreads toward the cuticle is _____. As the

condition matures, the discoloration becomes _____ .

23. A type of fungus infection caused when moisture is trapped between an unsanitized natural nail and products that are put over the natural nail, such as tips, wraps, gels, or acrylic nails,

is called _____ .

24. Describe how to identify nail mold in early stages.

_____

25. Describe how to identify advanced nail mold.

_____

26. Name two procedures to follow if a client has nail fungus or nail mold.

1. _____

2. _____

27. List the four safety precautions to follow when removing products from nails with fungus or mold.

1. _____

2. _____

3. _____

4. _____

_____

28. Identify four ways to avoid nail mold and nail fungus.

    1. _____

    2. _____

    3. _____

    4. _____

NAIL DISEASES

29. Name four signs of an infection.

    1. _____ 2. _____

    3. _____ 4. _____

30. When working with chemicals, a cosmetologist's hands and nails should be protected with

    _____ .

31. Matching: *Match the nail diseases on the left with their correct descriptions on the right.*

    ____ 1. onychocryptosis   A. periodic nail shedding

    ____ 2. athlete's foot   B. ringworm of the nails

    ____ 3. onychoptosis   C. ringworm of the foot

    ____ 4. onychophosis   D. brittle, split nails

    ____ 5. onychomycosis   E. swelling of the nail

    ____ 6. paronychia   F. nail disease

    ____ 7. onycholysis   G. a bluish colored nail

    ____ 8. onychogryposis   H. growth of horny epithelium in the nail bed

    ____ 9. onychia   I. infected and inflamed tissue surrounding

    ____ 10. onychophyma   the nail

    ____ 11. onychosis   J. white spots on the nail

                                  K. ingrown nails

                                  L. loosening of the nail

                                  M. inflamed nail matrix

                                  N. enlarged/increased nail curve

WORD REVIEW

agnail	irregularities	onycholysis
athlete's foot	keratin	onychomycosis
atrophy	leuconychia	onychophagy
blue nails	lunula	onychophosis
bruised nails	malformation	onychophyma
corrugations	mantle	onychoptosis
cuticle	matrix	onychorrhexis
depressions	nail bed	onychosis
disease	nail body	onyx
disorder	nail fungus	parasites
eggshell nails	nail grooves	paronychia
eponychium	nail mold	perionychium
free edge	nail root	plate
furrows	nail walls	pterygium
hangnail	onychatrophia	ringworm
hypertrophy	onychauxis	tinea unguium
hyponychium	onychia	vesicles
infection	onychocryptosis	wavy ridges
ingrown nail	onychogryposis	

THEORY OF MASSAGE

INTRODUCTION

1. List three reasons why massage is used.

   1. _____   2. _____

   3. _____

2. Massage involves the application of external _____ to the head and _____.

3. Six electrical appliances used in massage are:

   1. _____   2. _____

   3. _____   4. _____

   5. _____   6. _____

4. Your massage services are limited to the following body areas:

   1. _____   2. _____

   3. _____   4. _____

   5. _____   6. _____

   7. _____

5. It is important that you give massage with a firm, _____ touch.

6. To prevent drag or damage to the client's skin, apply cream or _____ to your hands.

7. The final massage results depend on the:

   1. _____

   2. _____

   3. _____

8. Direction of massage movement should be from muscle insertion toward its _____.

   The end of a muscle that is attached to a bone or tissue is the _____. The other end of

   a muscle (attached to another muscle or to a movable bone or joint) is the _____.

BASIC MANIPULATIONS USED IN MASSAGE

9. Identification Match: *Using the letters E, P, F, T, and V (as defined below), match the correct characteristics listed below with one of the massage manipulations.*

Key:

E=effleurage
P=petrissage
F=friction
T=tapotement or percussion
V=vibration

Characteristics:

_____   1. a light, continuous stroking movement

_____   2. squeeze, roll, or pinch

_____   3. the most stimulating massage movement

_____   4. "fulling" is one form of it

_____   5. no pressure is used

_____   6. chucking, rolling, and wringing are variations

_____   7. accomplished by rapid muscular contractions in your arms

_____   8. a kneading movement

_____   9. limit to a few seconds on any one spot

_____ 10. has soothing and relaxing effects

_____ 11. a shaking movement

_____ 12. influences circulation and glandular activity of the skin

_____ 13. invigorating movement for deep stimulation

_____ 14. tapping, slapping, and hacking movements

SAFETY PRECAUTIONS

10. Name the three health considerations that prevent your giving a massage.

1. _____   2. _____

3. _____

11. Why is massage harmful to clients with the health conditions named above?

_____

12. Vigorous massage should not be used on clients with _____.

PHYSIOLOGICAL EFFECTS OF MASSAGE

13. The three structures involved in massage are:

1. _____   2. _____

3. _____

14. Every muscle and nerve has a motor _____. You must consider these in massage

because they effect the underlying _____ of the face and neck.

15. Identify the names of motor nerve points on the illustration below.

1. _____

2. _____

3. _____

4. _____

5. _____

6. _____

16. The immediate effects of massage are first noticed on the _____.

17. In what four ways do the parts being massaged respond?

    1. _____   2. _____

    3. _____   4. _____

18. List seven benefits of massage.

    1. _____

    2. _____

    3. _____

    4. _____

    5. _____

    6. _____

    7. _____

19. If a client wants to relax, what type of manipulations should you use?

    1. _____

    2. _____

20. If you want to stimulate body tissues, you should use manipulations that are either:

    1. _____

    2. _____

21. Fatty tissues can be reduced by firm _____, or by fast, firm, and light _____

    movements over a fairly _____ period of time.

22. How often you give a facial or scalp massage depends on the following:

    1. _____   2. _____

    3. _____

23. As a general rule, normal skin or scalp can be kept in excellent condition with the help of a

    _____ massage.

WORD REVIEW

anatomy
chucking
circulation
digital
effleurage
electrical appliances
external
friction
fulling
heating caps

high-frequency current
insertion
manipulation
massage
motor point
muscle
origin
palmar
percussion

petrissage
physiology
rolling
steamers
tapotement
therapeutic lamps
vibration
vibrators
wringing

19

FACIALS

See *Milady's Standard Practical Workbook.*

FACIAL MAKEUP

INTRODUCTION

1. What is the main objective of a makeup application?

_____

_____

2. The four things you must consider when applying makeup are:

   1. _____   2. _____

   3. _____   4. _____

3. Using makeup allows you to create optical illusions with shadowing, _____,

   and _____.

PREPARATION FOR MAKEUP APPLICATION

4. If a client has both hair and makeup service, when should you do the makeup?

   1. _____

   2. _____

5. Remove products from their containers with either a _____ or

   _____.

6. Wash and _____ your hands before _____ the _____ face.

7. When selecting and applying makeup, be sure to have a well-lighted _____,

   and, when possible, check the makeup in _____.

COSMETICS FOR FACIAL MAKEUP

8. The most important makeup item is probably _____.

9. List four purposes of foundation.

   1. _____

   2. _____

   3. _____

   4. _____

10. What determines the selection of foundation color? _____

11. List ten foundation color classifications.

    1. _____   2. _____

    3. _____   4. _____

    5. _____   6. _____

    7. _____   8. _____

    9. _____   10. _____

12. When choosing a foundation color for light skin, choose a shade _____ than the natural skin tone. When choosing one for dark skin, choose one that _____ the natural skin tone. For a sallow skin, choose a _____ foundation. And, for a florid skin tone, choose a _____ foundation.

13. In order to see if the foundation color chosen will be appropriate on the client, place a small _____ on the client's _____.

14. The most widely used types of foundations are:

    1. _____   2. _____

15. Identification Match: *Using the letters CR, LQ, CA, ST, and BM (as defined below), match the correct characteristics listed below with one foundation type.*

Key:

CR=cream foundation

LQ=liquid foundation

CA=cake foundation

ST=stick foundation

BM=blemish masking creams/sticks

Characteristics:

_____ 1. adds color and gives a velvety look

_____ 2. gives the most natural look

_____ 3. may be applied before or after foundation

_____ 4. color suspended in a semi-liquid delicate, light oil

_____ 5. has a thick consistency

_____ 6. effective for oily skin

_____ 7. available in a range of colors to match skin tones

_____ 8. patted over a blemish before blending

_____ 9. formulated for normal, dry, and oily skin types

16. Name four purposes of face powders.

    1. _____

    2. _____

    3. _____

    4. _____

17. The two forms face powders come in are:

    1. _____   2. _____

18. For dry/normal skin, it is best to use a face powder of _____ or _____

    weight. Oily skin requires a face powder that is _____.

19. The three ways face powder should never look are:

    1. _____   2. _____

    3. _____

20. Face powders are applied _____ foundation by using a cotton _____ or

    _____. The powder helps to _____ the makeup.

21. What is the purpose of cheek color?

    _____

22. Cheek color should coordinate with the _____ color. During the day, cheek color should

    be less _____

23. Liquid cheek color should be applied _____ foundation, but _____ powdering
the face.

24. For dry and normal skin, _____ color is preferred.

25. Dry cheek color gives a _____ finish.

26. Brush-on cheek color is used to add _____ and to _____ the cheeks.

27. List three purposes of lip color.

    1. _____

    2. _____

    3. _____

28. Lip color must _____ be applied _____ from the container unless it belongs

    to _____. Remove the color from its container with a _____, then take it

    from the _____ with a _____.

29. To emphasize lip lines, you may choose to use a _____.

30. Eye colors, or _____, make eyes appear _____ and more

    _____.

31. There are _____ set rules for selection of eye makeup colors except they should enhance

    the _____ and be more _____ in daytime.

32. The four forms of eye shadows are:

    1. _____   2. _____

    3. _____   4. _____

33. The three forms of eyeliner are:

    1. _____ 2. _____

    3. _____

34. Eyeliners create a _____ on the eyelid close to the _____ to make the eyes

    appear _____ and the lashes _____.

35. Four reasons for using eyebrow pencils are:

    1. _____ 2. _____

    3. _____ 4. _____

36. Why do you have to use a fresh eyebrow pencil for each client?

    _____

37. The three forms mascara comes in are:

    1. _____ 2. _____

    3. _____

38. Mascara enhances natural _____, makes them appear _____ and

    _____, and can also be used to darken _____.

Also see *Milady's Standard Practical Workbook.*

WORD REVIEW

blemish masking cream/stick
blush
brush-on cheek color
cake foundation
cheek color
cream cheek color
cream foundation
dry cheek color
eye color

eye shadow
eyebrow pencil
eyeliner
face powder
foundation
fresh applicator
gloss
lip color
lipstick

liquid cheek color
liquid foundation
makeup
mascara
rouge
sanitized spatula
stick foundation
translucent powder

THE SKIN AND ITS DISORDERS

INTRODUCTION

1. The largest organ of the body is the _____.

2. If you have a thorough understanding of the skin, you can give clients advice on the care of their:

    1. _____   2. _____

    3. _____

3. List three characteristics of healthy skin.

    1. _____   2. _____

    3. _____

4. The skin's feel and appearance make up its _____, which, ideally, is smooth and fine

    _____.

5. The appendages of the skin are:

    1. _____   2. _____

    3. _____   4. _____

6. The part of the body where the skin is thinnest is on the _____; it is thickest on the

    palms and _____. A callus is a result of continuous _____ on one area.

HISTOLOGY OF THE SKIN

7. The two main divisions of the skin are the:

    1. _____   2. _____

8. The outermost layer of skin is the _____, which is also called the cuticle or

    _____.

9. A. Complete the list of the four layers, or stratums, of the epidermis.

    1. stratum co_____   2. stratum lu_____

    3. stratum gr_____   4. stratum ge_____

    B. Using numbers 1, 2, 3, and 4 from question #9A above, match them with the following characteristics.

    ___   1. cells are continually being shed
    ___   2. granular layer
    ___   3. formerly known as the stratum mucosum
    ___   4. clear layer
    ___   5. also called the horny layer
    ___   6. cells are almost dead
    ___   7. melanocytes are located here
    ___   8. transparent cells

10. Four other names for the dermis are:

1. _____ 2. _____

3. _____ 4. _____

11. The dermis is _____ times thicker than the _____. The two layers of the

dermis are the _____ and the _____ layer.

12. List three items found in the papillary layer.

1. _____ 2. _____

3. _____

13. Identify the parts of the skin illustrated below.

1. _____
2. _____
3. _____
4. _____
5. _____
6. _____
7. _____
8. _____
9. _____
10. _____
11. _____
12. _____
13. _____
14. _____
15. _____
16. _____
17. _____
18. _____
19. _____
20. _____
21. _____
22. _____
23. _____
24. _____
25. _____
26. _____
27. _____

14. List seven items found within the reticular layer.

1. _____ 2. _____

3. _____ 4. _____

5. _____ 6. _____

7. _____

15. The fatty layer below the dermis is called _____ tissue. Two other terms/

words used to describe this tissue are either _____ or _____ tissue.

16. Three purposes of this fat layer are:

    1. _____

    2. _____

    3. _____

17. What supplies nourishment to the skin?

    1. _____   2. _____

18. Three nerve fibers in the skin are:

    1. _____   2. _____

    3. _____

19. Nerve endings that deal with the sense of touch register the following six sensations:

    1. _____   2. _____

    3. _____   4. _____

    5. _____   6. _____

20. The part of the body where nerve endings are most abundant are the _____.

21. The pliability of the skin depends on the elasticity of the skin's _____ layer. The

    main characteristic of aged skin is its _____ of elasticity.

22. What two factors determine a person's skin color?

    1. _____

    2. _____

23. List two types of duct glands.

    1. _____   2. _____

24. Name four body parts that contain more numerous sweat glands than other parts.

    1. _____   2. _____

    3. _____   4. _____

25. The two purposes of the sweat glands are:

    1. _____   2. _____

26. Oil glands have ducts that open into the hair _____. The name of the oil this gland

    secretes is _____, which lubricates and softens the skin and _____.

27. When the duct becomes clogged due to hardened sebum, a _____ forms.

28. Identification Match: *Using the letters PR, SN, HR, EX, SC, and AB (as defined below), match the correct characteristics listed below with one of the six functions of the skin.*

    Key:

    PR=protection
    SN=sensation
    HR=heat regulation
    EX=excretion
    SC=secretion
    AB=absorption

    Characteristics:

    _____ 1. sebum lubricates and softens the skin

    _____ 2. happens to fatty materials through the hair follicles

    _____ 3. protects the body from the environment

    _____ 4. keeps the body from injury and bacterial invasion

    _____ 5. water takes salt and other chemicals with it

    _____ 6. stimulating nerves sends messages to the brain

    _____ 7. female hormones enter through the skin

    _____ 8. emotional stress can cause an increase in sebum flow

    _____ 9. responds to heat, cold, pain, touch, and pressure

    _____ 10. sebum renders the skin waterproof

    _____ 11. perspiration

    _____ 12. maintains a constant temperature of 98.6° F

DISORDERS OF THE SKIN

29. You should not serve a client who has an inflamed skin _____. Likewise, if you do

    not recognize this, or know what the problem is, refer the client to a _____.

30. Define the following terms.

    1. dermatology

    _____

    2. dermatologist

    _____

    3. pathology

    _____

    4. trichology

    _____

    5. etiology

    _____

    6. diagnosis

    _____

    7. prognosis

    _____

31. Define lesion.

_____

32. Name and describe two types of symptoms.

    1. _____

    2. _____

33. List the nine primary lesions. After each lesion, name or describe an example of each.

    1. _____

    2. _____

    3. _____

    4. _____

    5. _____

    6. _____

    7. _____

    8. _____

    9. _____

34. List the seven secondary lesions. After each lesion, name or describe an example of each.

    1. _____

    2. _____

    3. _____

    4. _____

    5. _____

    6. _____

    7. _____

35. Matching: *Match the terms on the left with their correct descriptions on the right.*

____ 1. congenital
        disease
____ 2. allergy
____ 3. infectious disease
____ 4. skin disease
____ 5. epidemic
____ 6. parasitic disease
____ 7. acute disease
____ 8. systemic disease
____ 9. disease
____ 10. seasonal disease
____ 11. inflammation
____ 12. pathogenic disease
____ 13. chronic disease
____ 14. venereal disease
____ 15. occupational disease

A. any departure from a normal
      state of health
B. primary lesions
C. long duration disease
D. due to certain kinds of employment
E. can be caused by faulty diet
F. present at birth
G. a sensitivity to normally harmless substances
H. influenced by the weather
I. caused by vegetable/animal parasites
J. any infection of the skin
K. produced by disease-causing bacteria
L. violent symptoms and short duration
M. acquired through sexual intercourse
N. caused by non-pathogenic bacteria
O. characterized by redness, pain, swelling, and heat
P. due to germs taken into the body by contact with a
      contaminated object or lesion
Q. an example is trichoptilosis
R. simultaneously attacks a large number of people
      living in a particular locality

36. The technical name for blackheads is _____, which are formed from hardened

    _____. They most commonly form on the face, _____, and _____

    and often occur between the ages of 13 and ____.

37. The technical name for a whitehead is _____, which is a disorder of the

    _____ gland.

38. Acne is a chronic, _____ disorder, and is also known as acne _____

    or acne _____. It should always be examined by a _____ before giving any
    salon service.

39. An oily or shiny skin condition is called _____. A condition of dry skin is known

    as _____.

40. An inflammation congestion of the cheeks and nose is _____.

41. A sebaceous cyst filled with sebum is called either steatoma or _____. It most

    commonly appears on the scalp, _____, and _____.

42. Foul-smelling perspiration is called _____. Lack of perspiration is called

    _____. Excessive perspiration is called _____.

43. Exposure to excessive heat may cause _____, commonly called prickly heat.

44. Matching: *Match the terms on the left with their correct descriptions on the right.*

    ____ 1. dermatitis   A.   many forms of dry or moist lesions

    ____ 2. naevus   B.   inflammatory skin condition

    ____ 3. eczema   C.   leucoderma affecting skin or hair

    ____ 4. keratoma   D.   small brownish spot

    ____ 5. tan   E.   fever blisters

    ____ 6. stains   F.   skin cancer

    ____ 7. leucoderma   G.   round, dry patches with silvery scales

    ____ 8. psoriasis   H.   callus

    ____ 9. verruca   I.   absence of melanin

    ____ 10. albinism   J.   abnormal brown skin patches

    ____ 11. herpes simplex   K.   liver spots

    ____ 12. melanotic sarcoma   L.   abnormal white patches

    ____ 13. vitiligo   M.   excessive exposure to the sun

    ____ 14. lentigenes   N.   absence of perspiration

    ____ 15. mole   O.   birthmark

    ____ 16. chloasma   P.   comedone

                                    Q.   wart

                                    R.   freckles

                                    S.   foul-smelling perspiration

45. People who specialize in skin care are professionally called _____.

46. Briefly define the following terms.

    1. rhytidectomy _____

    2. blepharoplasty _____

    3. chemical peeling _____

    4. rhinoplasty _____

    5. mentoplasty _____

    6. dermabrasion _____

    7. injectable fillers _____

    8. Retin-A™ _____

WORD REVIEW: THE SKIN

absorption	excretion	sebaceous gland
adipose tissue	fundus	sebum
arrector pili muscles	heat regulation	secretion
arteries	histologist	secretory nerve fibers
blepharoplasty	injectable fillers	sensation
capillaries	lymphatics	sensory nerve fibers
chemical peeling	melanocyte	stratum corneum
corium	mentoplasty	stratum germinativum
cutis	motor nerve fibers	stratum granulosum
derma	oil glands	stratum lucidum
dermabrasion	papillae	stratum mucosum
dermatologist	papillary layer	subcutaneous tissue
dermatology	pathology	subcutis
dermis	protection	suderiferous
diagnosis	reticular layer	sweat glands
elasticity	Retin-A™	tactile corpuscles
epidermis	rhinoplasty	trichology
esthetician	rhytidectomy	true skin
etiology		

WORD REVIEW: DISORDERS

acne	fissure	psoriasis
acute diseases	herpes simplex	pustule
albinism	hyperhydrosis	rosacea
allergy	infectious disease	scale
anhidrosis	inflammation	scar
asteatosis	keratoma	seasonal disease
bromidrosis	lentigines	seborrhea
bulla	lesion	skin disease
chloasma	leucoderma	stain/s
chronic disease	macule	steatoma
comedone	melanotic sarcoma	subjective symptoms
congenital disease	milia	systemic disease
contagious disease	miliaria rubra	tan
crust	mole	tubercle
cyst	naevus	tumor
dermatitis	objective symptoms	ulcer
diagnosis	occupational disease	venereal disease
disease	papule	verruca
eczema	parasitic disease	vesicle
epidemic	pathogenic disease	vitiligo
etiology	pathology	wheal
excoriation	prognosis	

REMOVING UNWANTED HAIR

INTRODUCTION

1. List three terms used to describe hair growth in unusual amounts or locations.

    1. _____   2. _____

    3. _____

2. Ancient Greek and Roman women removed their unwanted hair by using a method of

    _____.

3. The two types of hair removal are:

    1. _____   2. _____

PERMANENT METHODS OF HAIR REMOVAL

4. In 1875, Charles E. Michel devised the technique of _____. He used a direct

    electric current that is called _____. This technique decomposed the dermal

    _____ in order that hair could not grow back.

5. In 1924, Dr. H. Brodier developed _____, which used _____ frequency

    current. This method, in order to destroy the papilla, used _____ and was much faster
    than the galvanic process.

6. In 1945, the _____ method was developed. It was called this because it blended

    _____ current with low-intensity _____ shortwave current.

7. An unskilled electrologist could cause irreparable _____ to the skin.

8. The machine used in electrolysis is called a _____ machine.

9. List eight body areas that may be treated with electrolysis.

    1. _____   2. _____

    3. _____   4. _____

    5. _____   6. _____

    7. _____   8. _____

10. List three body areas that should NOT be treated with electrolysis.

    1. _____   2. _____

    3. _____

11. Name five factors that may cause unwanted hair growth.

1. _____   2. _____

3. _____   4. _____

5. _____

12. Another name for the shortwave method is the _____ method.

Also see *Milady's Standard Practical Workbook.*

WORD REVIEW

alternating current	electrolysis	hypertrichosis
blend method	epilator	permanent removal
blended galvanic current	Federal Communications	*rusma*
depilatory	Commission	shortwave machine
dermal papilla	galvanic	superfluous hair
direct current	high-frequency current	temporary removal
electrology	hirsuties	thermolysis method

CELLS, ANATOMY, AND PHYSIOLOGY

INTRODUCTION

1. List four parts of which the human organism is made.

    1. _____   2. _____

    3. _____   4. _____

2. Cellular parts are composed of _____.

CELLS

3. The basic units of all living things are _____.

4. Cells are made up of _____.

5. List the five main parts of a cell.

    1. _____   2. _____

    3. _____   4. _____

    5. _____

6. Identify the parts of the cell illustrated below.

   1. _____

   2. _____

   3. _____

   4. _____

   5. _____

   6. _____

7. Which part of a cell contains food materials? _____

8. Which two parts of a cell affect its reproduction?

    1. _____   2. _____

9. What cell part encloses the protoplasm? _____

10. What does a cell need in order to grow?

1. _____   2. _____

3. _____   4. _____

5. _____

11. Metabolism is the chemical process by which cells are nourished and supplied with energy.

The process of building up larger molecules from smaller ones is called _____.

The process of breaking down larger molecules into smaller ones is known as _____.

12. The body stores food, water, and oxygen during _____ and releases energy

during _____.

13. If molecules of energy are not used, they turn into _____.

TISSUES

14. Tissues are groups of _____ of the same kind.

15. List five tissue types.

1. _____   2. _____

3. _____   4. _____

5. _____

ORGANS

16. Structures designed to accomplish a specific _____ are organs.

17. List the six most important body organs.

1. _____   2. _____

3. _____   4. _____

5. _____   6. _____

SYSTEMS

18. Groups of _____ that cooperate for a common purpose are systems.

INTRODUCTION TO ANATOMY AND PHYSIOLOGY

19. Define anatomy.

_____

20. Define physiology.

_____

21. Define histology.

_____

THE SKELETAL SYSTEM

22. What is the hardest tissue of the body? _____

23. The scientific study of bones, their structure, and their functions is called _____.

24. Name five functions of bones.

    1. _____

    2. _____

    3. _____

    4. _____

    5. _____

25. Of what two types of matter is bone composed?

    1. One-third _____ matter

    2. Two-thirds _____ matter

26. Name the two parts into which the skull is divided.

    1. _____   2. _____

27. Name eight bones of the cranium.

    1. _____   2. _____

    3. _____   4. _____

    5. _____   6. _____

28. Name fourteen bones of the face.

    1. _____   2. _____

    3. _____   4. _____

    5. _____   6. _____

    7. _____   8. _____

29. Identify the bones of the head, face and neck illustrated below.

1. _____

2. _____

3. _____

4. _____

5. _____

6. _____

7. _____

8. _____

9. _____

10. _____

11. _____

12. _____

13. _____

14. _____

15. _____

16. _____

17. _____

30. What is the name of the bone commonly called the "Adam's apple?" _____

31. What is the thorax?

_____

_____

32. The twelve ribs on each side are called _____; the breastbone is called the

_____.

33. Name the three bones in the arm.

1. _____   2. _____

3. _____

34. What are the wrist bones called? _____.

35. The palm has five bones called _____, and the fingers, or _____, have

a total of fourteen _____ in them.

36. Identify the bones of the arm and hand illustrated below.

1. _____

2. _____

3. _____

4. _____

5. _____

1. _____

2. _____

3. _____

4. _____

5. _____

THE MUSCULAR SYSTEM

37. The study of the structure, functions, and diseases of muscles is called _____.

38. There are over _____ muscles in the body and they comprise between _____ percent of human body weight.

39. The three kinds of muscular tissue are:

1. _____   2. _____

3. _____

40. The fixed muscle attachment is called the _____, and the movable muscle attachment

is called the _____. The middle part is known as the _____.

41. Name seven methods used to stimulate muscles.

1. _____   2. _____

3. _____   4. _____

5. _____   6. _____

7. _____

42. Pressure in massage is usually directed from the _____ to the _____.

43. Name the two parts of the epicranius.

1. _____   2. _____

44. Which part lifts the eyebrows? _____

45. Identify the muscles illustrated below.

1. _____

2. _____

3. _____

4. _____

5. _____

6. _____

7. _____

8. _____

9. _____

10. _____

11. _____

12. _____

13. _____

14. _____

15. _____

16. _____

17. _____

18. _____

19. _____

20. _____

21. _____

22. _____

23. _____

46. Matching: *Match the terms on the left with their correct descriptions on the right.*

_____ 1. caninus

_____ 2. orbicularis oris

_____ 3. mentalis

_____ 4. orbicularis oculi

_____ 5. auricularis superior

_____ 6. quadratus labii superioris

_____ 7. masseter

_____ 8. zygomaticus

_____ 9. corrugator

_____ 10. auricularis anterior

_____ 11. triangularis

_____ 12. sternocleidomastoid

_____ 13. risorius

_____ 14. platysma

_____ 15. procerus

_____ 16. auricularis posterior

_____ 17. buccinator

A. compresses and contracts the lips, as in kissing or whistling

B. muscle in front of the ear

C. expels air between the lips, as in blowing

D. raises the arm

E. allows the closing of the eyes

F. depresses the lower jaw and lip, as in expressing sadness

G. muscle behind the ear

H. causes wrinkling of the chin, as in doubt/displeasure

I. causes wrinkles across the bridge of the nose

J. draws the corner of the mouth out and back, as in grinning

K. straightens the fingers

L. draws back the upper lip and elevates the nostrils, as in expressing distaste

M. rotates and bends the head, as in nodding

N. muscle used for frowning

O. muscle above the ear

P. a chewing muscle

Q. raises the angle of the mouth, as in snarling

R. draws down corner of mouth

S. elevates the lip, as in laughing

47. To rotate the shoulder blade and control swinging movements of the arm, you use the

_____ and _____ muscles.

48. The three muscles of the shoulder and upper arm are:

1. _____   2. _____

3. _____

49. Name the four muscles of the forearm.

1. _____   2. _____

3. _____   4. _____

50. Name three muscles found in the hand.

1. _____   2. _____

3. _____

THE NERVOUS SYSTEM

51. The branch of anatomy that deals with the nervous system and its disorders is called

_____.

52. List the three main divisions of the nervous system.

1. _____

2. _____

3. _____

53. The nervous system that controls all body movements and facial expressions is the

_____.

54. The nervous system that carries messages to and from the central nervous system is the

_____.

55. The nervous system that has two divisions—the sympathetic and parasympathetic systems—

is the _____.

56. The central power station of the body, and also the largest mass of nerve tissue in the body,

is the _____ , which weighs between _____ and _____ ounces.

57. What is the primary structural unit of the nervous system? _____

58 What are the names of the types of nerves that carry messages concerning touch, cold, taste,

hearing, sight, pain, heat, and pressure to the brain? _____

59. What type of nerve carries impulses from the brain to the muscles?

_____

60. Which nerve type has the ability to both send and receive messages? _____

61. An automatic response to a stimulus that involves the movement of an impulse is called a

_____.

62. The chief nerve of the face, and the largest of the cranial nerves, is known by the following
three terms:

1. _____   2. _____

3. _____

63. List eight branches of the fifth cranial nerve that are affected by massage.

1. _____   2. _____

3. _____   4. _____

5. _____   6. _____

7. _____   8. _____

64. List the six most important branches of the seventh cranial nerve.

    1. _____   2. _____

    3. _____   4. _____

    5. _____   6. _____

65. The eleventh cranial nerve affects the muscles of the neck and _____.

66. What is the name of the nerve that affects the scalp as far up as the top of the head?

    _____

67. What is the name of the nerve that is located at the side of the neck and affects the neck as far

    down as the breastbone? _____

68. List the four main nerves of the arm and hand.

    1. _____   2. _____

    3. _____   4. _____

69. Identify the nerves in the head, face, and neck illustrated below.

    1. _____
    2. _____
    3. _____
    4. _____
    5. _____
    6. _____
    7. _____
    8. _____
    9. _____
    10. _____
    11. _____
    12. _____
    13. _____
    14. _____
    15. _____
    16. _____
    17. _____
    18. _____

70. Identify the nerves of the arm and hand illustrated below.

1. _____

2. _____

3. _____

4. _____

THE CIRCULATORY SYSTEM

71. Another name for the circulatory system is the _____ system.

72. The two divisions of this system are:

   1. _____   2. _____

73. The heart is enclosed in a membrane called the _____. At normal resting rate,

   the heart beats _____ to _____ times per minute.

74. The four valves of the heart are the:

   1. _____   2. _____

   3. _____   4. _____

75. Identify the parts of the heart illustrated below.

1. _____
2. _____
3. _____
4. _____
5. _____
6. _____
7. _____
8. _____
9. _____
10. _____
11. _____
12. _____
13. _____
14. _____
15. _____
16. _____
17. _____
18. _____
19. _____
20. _____
21. _____
22. _____
23. _____
24. _____

76. Veins carry blood _____ the heart, while arteries carry blood _____ from it.

77. Blood is defined as _____. An
     adult has between _____ and _____ pints of blood.

78. The two systems that circulate blood are:
     1. _____   2. _____

79. Red corpuscles carry _____ to the cells; white corpuscles _____ disease-
     causing germs. The fluid in which they grow is called _____.

80. In very simple terms, write down five functions of blood.

    1. _____

    2. _____

    3. _____

    4. _____

    5. _____

81. A medium of exchange, trading nutritive materials to the cells for waste products, is a

    colorless, watery fluid called _____.

82. Which artery supplies blood to the face, mouth, and nose? _____

83. Identify the arteries of the head, face, and neck illustrated below.

1. _____

2. _____

3. _____

4. _____

5. _____

6. _____

7. _____

8. _____

9. _____

10. _____

11. _____

12. _____

13. _____

14. _____

15. _____

16. _____

84. Which artery supplies muscles, skin, and scalp? _____

85. The two principal veins on each side of the neck are the:

    1. _____   2. _____

86. Identify the arteries of the hand and arm illustrated below.

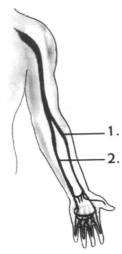

1. _____

2. _____

1.
2.

THE ENDOCRINE SYSTEM

87. Specialized organs that vary in size and function are known as _____. They are

controlled by the body's _____ system.

88. The two sets of glands are the:

1. _____   2. _____

THE EXCRETORY SYSTEM

89. List the five parts of the body included in the excretory system.

1. _____   2. _____

3. _____   4. _____

5. _____

THE RESPIRATORY SYSTEM

90. The muscle that controls breathing is known as the _____. Two spongy tissues

that take in air are the _____.

91. Oxygen is absorbed during _____, while carbon dioxide is expelled during

_____. If a person does not get any _____ every few minutes, he/she may
die.

92. Breathing through the _____ is healthier than breathing through the mouth because

bacteria are caught by the nasal _____.

THE DIGESTIVE SYSTEM

93. The digestive system changes food into _____ form. Digestion starts in the _____ and is completed in the _____. The complete process takes about _____ hours.

94. Define digestive enzymes.

_____

WORD REVIEW: GENERAL

anabolism	endocrine system	nervous system
anatomy	epithelial tissue	nucleus
catabolism	excretory system	organs
cell membrane	histology	physiology
cells	integumentary system	protoplasm
centrosome	liquid tissue	reproductive system
circulatory system	metabolism	respiratory system
connective tissue	muscular system	skeletal system
cytoplasm	muscular tissue	systems
digestive system	nerve tissue	tissues

WORD REVIEW: SKELETAL SYSTEM

bone	mandible	shoulder
carpus	maxillae	skull
cervical vertebrae	metacarpus	sphenoid
cranium	nasal	sternum
digits	occipital	temporal
ethmoid	os	thoracic vertebrae
fingers	osteology	thorax
frontal	palatine	turbinal
girdle	palm	ulna
humerus	parietal	vomer
hyoid	phalanges	wrist
lacrimal	radius	zygomatic

WORD REVIEW: MUSCULAR SYSTEM

abductor	frontalis	platysma
adductor	insertion	procerus
aponeurosis	latissimus dorsi	pronators
auricularis anterior	masseter	quadratus labii inferioris
auricularis posterior	mentalis	quadratus labii superioris
auricularis superior	myology	risorius
belly	non-striated	serratus anterior
biceps	occipitalis	sternocleidomastoid
buccinator	occipito-frontalis	striated
caninus	opponent	supinators
cardiac	orbicularis oculi	temporalis
corrugator	orbicularis oris	trapezius
deltoid	origin	triangularis
epicranius	pectoralis major	triceps
extensors	pectoralis minor	zygomaticus
flexors		

WORD REVIEW: NERVOUS SYSTEM

afferent nerves
auriculo-temporal nerve
autonomic nervous system
axon
axon terminal
brain
buccal nerve
cerebro-spinal nervous system
cervical cutaneous nerve
cervical nerve
cutaneous colli nerve
dendrites
digital nerve
efferent nerves
eleventh (accessory) cranial
  nerve (spinal branch)
fifth cranial nerve
greater auricular nerve

greater occipital nerve
infra-orbital nerve
infra-trochlear nerve
mandibular nerve
maxillary
median nerve
mental nerve
mixed nerves
motor nerves
nasal nerve
nerve cell
nerves
neurology
neuron
ophthalmic
parasympathetic nervous
  system
peripheral nervous system

posterior auricular nerve
radical nerve
reflex
sensory nerves
seventh (facial)
  cranial nerve
smaller occipital nerve
spinal cord
supra-orbital nerve
supra-trochlear nerve
sympathetic nervous
  system
temporal nerve
trifacial nerve
trigeminal nerve
ulnar nerve
zygomatic nerve

WORD REVIEW: CIRCULATORY SYSTEM

angular artery
anterior auricular artery
arteries
atria
auricle
blood
blood platelets
blood-vascular system
capillaries
common carotid
  arteries
external jugular
facial artery
frontal artery
general circulation
heart

inferior labial artery
infra-orbital artery
internal jugular
lacteals
left atrium
left ventricle
leucocytes
lymph
lymph-vascular system
lymphatic system
middle temporal artery
occipital artery
parietal artery
pericardium
plasma

posterior auricular artery
pulmonary circulation
red corpuscles
right atrium
right ventricle
submental artery
superficial temporal artery
superior labial artery
supra-orbital artery
systemic circulation
transverse facial artery
vagus
vascular system
veins
white corpuscles

WORD REVIEW: ENDOCRINE SYSTEM

duct glands
ductless glands

endocrine glands
exocrine glands

glands

WORD REVIEW: EXCRETORY SYSTEM

kidneys
large intestine

liver
lungs

skin

WORD REVIEW: RESPIRATORY SYSTEM

abdominal
carbon dioxide
diaphragm

exhalation
inhalation
lungs

oxygen
respiratory

WORD REVIEW: DIGESTIVE SYSTEM

digestion
digestive enzymes

enzymes
esophagus

pharynx
soluble

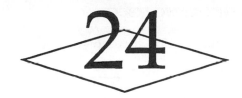

ELECTRICITY AND LIGHT THERAPY

ELECTRICITY

1. Define electricity.

   _____

2. The movement of electricity along a conductor is an electric _____ .

3. A substance that permits electric current to pass through it is a _____ .

   List seven examples of objects that allow this passage.

   1. _____   2. _____
   3. _____   4. _____
   5. _____   6. _____
   7. _____

4. A substance that resists the passage of electricity is known as either a _____

   or an _____ . List six examples of objects that resist this passage.

   1. _____   2. _____
   3. _____   4. _____
   5. _____   6. _____

5. Why is an electric wire considered to be composed of both of these (number 3 and number 4 above)?

   _____

6. Identification Match: *Using the letters DC and AC (as defined below), match the correct characteristics listed below with one type of current.*

   Key:

   DC=direct current
   AC=alternating current

   Characteristics:
   - _____ 1. constant, even-flowing current
   - _____ 2. produces a mechanical action
   - _____ 3. travels in one direction
   - _____ 4. a flashlight uses it
   - _____ 5. a plugged-in hair dryer uses it
   - _____ 6. a rapid and interrupted current
   - _____ 7. produces a chemical reaction
   - _____ 8. flows in one, then the opposite direction
   - _____ 9. a wall socket has this current
   - _____ 10. is generated by a battery

7. To change direct current into alternating current, you use a _____. To change alternating current into direct current, use a _____.

8. Matching: *Match the terms on the left with their correct descriptions on the right.*

___ 1. circuit breaker   A. safety device that prevents overheating of wires

___ 2. milliampere   B. equals 1,000 watts

___ 3. volt   C. measures current resistance

___ 4. kilowatt   D. unit that measures current pressure

___ 5. fuse   E. 1/10,000 part of an ampere

___ 6. watt   F. unit measuring how much energy is used in
                               one second
___ 7. amp/ampere

___ 8. ohm   G. 1/1,000 part of an ampere

                                                      H. measures the amount of current running
                               through a wire

                                                      I. measures wire length

                                                      J. a switch device that has largely replaced fuses

                                                      K. equals 10,000 watts

9. What may happen if you are careless when making electrical connections, or if you don't check for the right current amount? _____.

ELECTROTHERAPY

10. Define wall plate.

_____

_____.

11. What is the type of facial called that uses a wall plate? _____

12. List four types of modalities.

1. _____   2. _____

3. _____   4. _____.

13. What conducts the electric current from the machine to the client's skin? _____. It is usually made out of:

1. _____   2. _____

3. _____

14. Polarity is the negative or _____ state of electric current.

15. The most commonly used modality is the _____ current. A positive electrode is called an _____, has a _____ color, and is marked with either a "P" or _____ sign. A negative electrode is called a _____, has a _____ color, and is marked with either an "N" or _____ sign.

16. A positive pole _____ the pores, _____ blood supply, and hardens/firms tissues. On the other hand, a negative pole _____ the pores, _____ blood supply, and softens tissues.

17. The electrode to be used on the area to be treated is the _____ electrode. The client may hold the other electrode, which is called the _____ electrode.

18. Matching: *Match the terms on the left with their correct descriptions on the right.*

___ 1. faradic current	A. positive pole pulls positively charged substances into the skin
___ 2. phoresis	
___ 3. disincrustation	B. softens grease deposits in hair follicles and pores
___ 4. sinusoidal current	C. stimulates hair removal
___ 5. cataphoresis	D. forces chemical solutions into unbroken skin
___ 6. anaphoresis	E. has negative effects on the skin
___ 7. indirect method	F. stimulates hair growth
___ 8. direct method	G. negative pole pushes negatively charged substances into the skin
	H. two felt-tipped electrodes are used
	I. greater stimulation and deeper penetration than faradic current
	J. wear an ankle protector
	K. wear a wrist electrode

19. A high frequency, or _____ current uses a _____ rate of oscillation, or vibration. It is also called the _____ ray. Its primary action is _____ producing, or thermal, and there are no _____ contractions.

20. List four conditions that Tesla current may improve.

1. _____   2. _____

3. _____   4. _____

21. The facial electrode's shape is _____, and the scalp electrode is shaped like a _____.

22. List three methods for using Tesla current.

1. _____   2. _____

3. _____

23. List six benefits of Tesla current.

1. _____   2. _____

3. _____   4. _____

5. _____   6. _____

24. Matching: *Match the terms on the left with their correct descriptions on the right.*

___ 1. heating cap	A. used in plain manicure
___ 2. electric chair hair dryer	B. reduces processing time
___ 3. steamer	C. contains 8% of natural sunlight
___ 4. electric oil heater	D. produces moist, uniform heat
___ 5. electrically heated curling irons	E. increases processing time
	F. has an adjustable hood
___ 6. processing machine	G. oil is injected into its barrel
___ 7. hand dryer	H. used in oil manicure
	I. used to recondition dry, brittle hair
	J. delivers hot, medium, and cold air

LIGHT THERAPY

25. Define light therapy. _____

26. The _____ is the basic source of light rays. Invisible infrared rays make up _____ percent of natural sunlight, while ultraviolet rays make up _____ percent. Infrared rays produce _____; ultraviolet rays produce both chemical and _____ reactions.

27. List the colors of the rays of the visible spectrum.

    1. _____   2. _____
    3. _____   4. _____
    5. _____   6. _____
    7. _____

28. We can produce light rays by using a _____ lamp.

29. The client's eyes should always be _____ during light therapy. To do so, you may saturate a cotton pad with either boric acid solution, _____, or _____. Likewise, the cosmetologist should wear safety _____ when performing light therapy.

30. Which rays produce the most heat? _____

31. Briefly list six effects of infrared rays.

    1. _____
    2. _____
    3. _____
    4. _____
    5. _____
    6. _____

32. Two other names for ultraviolet rays are:

    1. _____   2. _____

33. Identification Match: *Using the letters UVA, UVB, and UVC, match the correct characteristics listed below with one type of ultraviolet ray.*

    _____ 1. furthest away from the visible spectrum
    _____ 2. in the middle of the UV range
    _____ 3. used in tanning booths
    _____ 4. most germicidal and chemical
    _____ 5. causes most burning to the skin
    _____ 6. therapeutic rays
    _____ 7. closest to the visible spectrum
    _____ 8. causes premature aging and wrinkling

34. Ultraviolet rays can penetrate up to _____ feet below water and approximately _____ percent can penetrate through a wet T-shirt.

35. List seven benefits of ultraviolet rays.

    1. _____   2. _____

    3. _____   4. _____

    5. _____   6. _____

    7. _____

36. List four disadvantages of ultraviolet rays.

    1. _____   2. _____

    3. _____   4. _____

37. Identification Match: *Using the letters W, B, and R (as defined below), match the correct characteristics listed below with one of the light rays.*

    Key:

    W=white light
    B=blue light
    R=red light

    Characteristics:

    ____ 1. used on bare, oily skin

    ____ 2. deepest penetrating of the visible spectrum

    ____ 3. does not penetrate

    ____ 4. relieves pain around nerve centers

    ____ 5. used on dry skin with creams/oils

    ____ 6. a combination light

WORD REVIEW

accelerating machine
actinic ray
active electrode
alternating current (AC)
amp
ampere
anaphoresis
anode
blue light
cataphoresis
cathode
circuit breaker
cold ray
complete circuit
   of electricity
conductor
converter
direct current (DC)
direct method
direct surface application
disincrustation
electric chair hair dryer
electric current
electric oil heater
electric wire

electrically heated
   curling iron
electricity
electrode
electrotherapy
faradic current
fuse
galvanic current
general electrification
hand dryer
heating cap
inactive electrode
indirect method
indirect surface
   application
infrared rays
insulator
invisible spectrum/
   light rays
kilowatt
light therapy
milliampere
modalities
negative
non-conductor

ohm
phoresis
polarity
positive
processing machine
rectifier
red light
sinusoidal current
steamer
Tesla high-frequency
   current
therapeutic lamp
ultraviolet rays
UVA
UVB
UVC
vaporizer
vibrator
violet ray
visible spectrum/
   light rays
volt
wall plate
watt
white light

Date _____
Rating _____
Text Pages 545–580

CHEMISTRY

THE SCIENCE OF CHEMISTRY

1. Define chemistry.

   _____

   _____.

2. The chemistry branch that deals with the presence of carbon is _____ chemistry. If

   no carbon is present, the branch of chemistry involved is _____ chemistry.

MATTER

3. Define matter.

   _____

   _____.

4. The basic _____ of all matter is an element. There are more than _____ known elements.

5. The smallest particle of an element is an _____. If two or more of these are joined

   chemically, a _____ is formed.

6. Define compound.

   _____

   _____.

7. List the four classes of compounds.

   1. _____ 2. _____

   3. _____ 4. _____

8. Define mixture.

   _____

9. What type of change occurs when ice melts into a liquid? _____

10. What type of change occurs when you mix hydrogen peroxide into a para dye?

   _____

11. List five physical property characteristics.

    1. _____ 2. _____

    3. _____ 4. _____

    5. _____

12. Define chemical properties _____

13. List two other names for chemical properties.

    1. _____ 2. _____

14. Matching: *Match the terms on the left with their correct descriptions on the right.*

    ____ 1. hydrogen   A.   readily releases oxygen

    ____ 2. combustion   B.   found in ammonia and nitrate forms

    ____ 3. oxidizing agent   C.   solution with pH higher than 7

    ____ 4. reducing agent   D.   slow rate of reaction

    ____ 5. oxygen   E.   pH of 7

    ____ 6. acid   F.   the substance that attracts

    ____ 7. hydrogen peroxide   G.   the least abundant element

    ____ 8. nitrozine paper   H.   colorless, odorless, and tasteless gas

    ____ 9. alkaline   I.   solution with pH less than 7

    ____ 10. slow oxidation   J.   the most abundant element

    ____ 11. nitrogen   K.   destroys pH

                               L.   3 percent solution is used as an antiseptic

                               M.   lighting a match, for example

                               N.   measures pH

CHEMISTRY OF WATER

15. The chemical symbol for water is _____.

16. Water is the most abundant and important _____ on the _____. About

    _____ percent of the human body and _____ percent of the earth's _____

    are water.

17. Fresh water is purified by sedimentation and _____. To kill bacteria, small

    amounts of _____ are added. Boiling water at a temperature of _____ degrees
    Fahrenheit will also kill most microbic life.

18. Protons are positive charges and electrons are _____ charges.

CHEMISTRY OF SHAMPOOS

19. What ingredient do most shampoos have in common? _____

20. The cleansing agent in shampoos is called either a base _____or a base

    _____.

21. Identification Match: *Using the letters AN, CA, NO, and AM (as defined below), match the correct characteristics listed below with one base surfactant.*

    Key:

    AN=anionics
    CA=catonics
    NO=nonionics
    AM=ampholytes

    Characteristics:

    _____ 1. contain quats

    _____ 2. one is cocamide

    _____ 3. one is sodium lauryl sulfate

    _____ 4. used in baby shampoos

    _____ 5. versatile, stable, and resists shrinkage

    _____ 6. the most commonly used detergents

    _____ 7. included in dandruff shampoos

    _____ 8. conducive to hair manageability

22. Water is attracted by the _____ surfactant end, and oil is attracted by the

    _____ end.

23. Matching: *Match the terms on the left with their correct descriptions on the right.*

    ___ 1. humectant   A. hydrolized protein replaces keratin
    ___ 2. polymer   B. composed of 32 amino acids
    ___ 3. moisturizer   C. absorbs and holds moisture
    ___ 4. pack   D. drying to the hair
    ___ 5. instant conditioner E. composed of 23 amino acids
    ___ 6. protein   F. has a heavy cream base conditioner
                              G. left on the hair a short time
                              H. a solid or gas
                              I. 10–20 minute application time

PERMANENT WAVING

24. Hair is made of the protein _____ and has the following three layers:

    1. _____ 2. _____

    3. _____

25. Each amino acid is joined to another _____ bond. List the three bonds.

    1. _____ 2. _____

    3. _____

26. In perming, the disulfide bonds in the _____ layer must be broken and

    _____. Breaking the bonds is both a physical and _____ action.

27. The pH range of a neutralizer is between _____ and _____. List three main active ingredients that are used in neutralizers.

    1. _____   2. _____

    3. _____

28. List two types of chemical hair relaxers.

    1. _____   2. _____

THE CHEMISTRY OF HAIRCOLORING

29. Identification Match: Using *the letters TC, SP, OX, VT, MD, CD, and CR (as defined below), match the correct characteristics listed below with one of the haircolor chemicals.*

Key:

TC=temporary haircolors
SP=semi-permanent tints
OX=oxidation tints
VT=vegetable tints
MD=metallic dyes
CD=compound dyes
CR=color removers

Characteristics:

_____   1. another name is aniline derivative tint

_____   2. lawsone is present

_____   3. designed to last three to four weeks

_____   4. reacts adversely with oxidation solutions

_____   5. color molecules have lowest molecular weight

_____   6. also called certified colors

_____   7. two types are oil-based and dye solvents

_____   8. logwood, indigo, chamomile, and henna are used

_____   9. diffuses artificial color molecules

_____   10. coats the outside of the hair

_____   11. make up a small portion of the home haircoloring market

_____   12. only some penetration into the cortex

_____   13. an example is compound henna

_____   14. color molecules have greatest molecular weight

_____   15. used to remove color buildup

_____   16. examples are lead, silver, and copper

_____   17. can coat the hair unevenly

_____   18. traditional and polymer are two types

_____   19. composed of a base and couplers

_____   20. combination of vegetable and metallic dyes

30. What causes hair to lighten? _____

31. Identification Match: *Using the letters OB, CB, PB, TO, and CF (as defined below), match the correct characteristics listed below with one color product.*

    Key:

    OB=oil or liquid bleach
    CB=cream bleach
    PB=powder bleach
    TO=toners
    CF=color fillers

    Characteristics:

    _____ 1. protinators or activators are added

    _____ 2. contain no oil or conditioner

    _____ 3. contain sulfonated oils

    _____ 4. dye load is less than on a tint

    _____ 5. gentle enough to use on scalp, yet can lighten to pastels

    _____ 6. create a base to which tint molecules can attach

    _____ 7. contain dry ammonia

    _____ 8. equalize porosity

    _____ 9. mildest bleach

    _____ 10. designed for pre-lightened hair

    _____ 11. have an average pH of 10.

    _____ 12. cannot be applied to the scalp

    _____ 13. some have turkey feathers or cattle hooves

    _____ 14. have the least amount of lightening action

    _____ 15. pale, delicate shades

COSMETIC CHEMISTRY

32. Matching: *Match the terms on the left with their correct descriptions on the right.*

    ____ 1. concentrated solution   A. solidified in a mold

    ____ 2. solute   B. ammonia is a by-product

    ____ 3. emulsion   C. dissolves into liquid and forms a solution

    ____ 4. miscible

    ____ 5. O/W emulsions   D. nonmixable

    ____ 6. powders   E. less solute and more solvent

    ____ 7. ointments   F. mix of two types of matter

    ____ 8. pastes   G. cream rouge is an example

    ____ 9. dilute solution   H. to make them, mixing and sifting are used

    ____ 10. soaps   I. oil droplets in a water base

    ____ 11. saturated solution   J. mixable

    ____ 12. mucilages   K. glycerine is a by-product

    ____ 13. solution   L. aerosol container

    ____ 14. W/O emulsions   M. will not take any more solute

____ 15. immiscible

____ 16. suspension

____ 17. solvent

____ 18. sticks

N.   is able to dissolve another substance

O.   prepared with a colloidal mill

P.   grain or ethyl are types

Q.   mixtures that do not separate

R.   lard, petrolatum, and wax are used

S.   water droplets in oil base

T.   more solute and less solvent

U.   hair setting lotion, for example

33. Matching: *Match the terms on the left with their correct descriptions on the right.*

____ 1. alcohol

____ 2. alum

____ 3. ammonia water

____ 4. boric acid

____ 5. ethyl methacrylate

____ 6. formaldehyde

____ 7. glycerine

____ 8. petrolatum

____ 9. phenylenediamine

____ 10. potassium

____ 11. quats in water

____ 12. sodium

____ 13. sodium carbonate

____ 14. witch hazel

____ 15. zinc oxide

A.   used in sculptured nails

B.   Vaseline or petroleum jelly

C.   from *Hamamelis virginiana* leaves and twigs

D.   quaternary ammonium compounds

E.   washing soda

F.   found in baby powder, eye creams, and soaps

G.   dishwashing soap

H.   decomposed oils, fats, or molasses

I.   grain or ethyl

J.   heavy white powder that is insoluble

K.   baking soda bicarbonate

L.   uses a colloidal mill

M.   stops bleeding

N.   derived from coal tar

O.   used as an embalming solution

P.   deodorant soap

Q.   ammonia gas dissolved in water

R.   caustic potash

34. What type of soap contains a bactericide for odors? _____

35. A soap made for delicate facial tissues is a _____.

36. What type of soaps are designed to treat problems such as acne? _____

37. A preparation for the temporary removal of superfluous hair is called a _____.

38. A tool that pulls hair out of the follicle is called an _____.

39. List four cream categories.

1. _____   2. _____

3. _____   4. _____

40. List six types of lotions.

1. _____   2. _____

3. _____   4. _____

5. _____   6. _____

41. Briefly list four qualities of a good face powder.

1. _____ 2. _____

3. _____ 4. _____

42. Two types of foundations are:

1. _____ 2. _____

43. The primary ingredient in lipsticks is _____.

44. A product used for theatrical purposes is _____.

45. What do hair dressings give to the hair? _____

46. What do styling aids give to the hair? _____

47. Hair spray is used to _____ the finished style.

WORD REVIEW

acids	greasepaint	petrolatum
alkalies	hardness	phenylenediamine
alum	humectant	physical change
ampholytic	hydrogen	polymers
amphoteric	hydrogen bond	potassium hydroxide
anionic	hydrophilic end	powders
atom	immiscible	pure hydrogen peroxide
base surfactant/detergent	inorganic chemistry	quats
boric acid	lawsone	reducing agent
cationic	lipophilic end	salts
chemical change/reaction	liquids	saturated solution
chemistry	lotions	soaps
colloidal mill	matter	sodium bicarbonate
color	miscible	sodium bromide
combustion	mixtures	sodium carbonate
compound	MOH Hardness Scale	sodium perborate
concentrated solution	molecule	solids
creams	mucilages	solute
density	nitrogen	solutions
depilatories	nitrozene paper	solvent
dilute solution	nonionic	specific gravity
disulfide bonds	oil-in-water-emulsions	sticks
element	ointments	sulfur bond
emulsions	organic chemistry	suspensions
epilators	oxides	volatile
ethyl methacrylate	oxidizing agents	water-in-oil emulsions
formaldehyde	oxygen packs	witch hazel
gases	pastes	zinc oxide
glycerine	peptide bond	

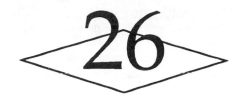

THE SALON BUSINESS

INTRODUCTION

1. List six topics that you must have knowledge of in order to be a salon owner and/or manager.

   1. _____   2. _____

   3. _____   4. _____

   5. _____   6. _____

WHAT YOU SHOULD KNOW ABOUT OPENING A SALON

2. A good location has a _____ large enough to support the salon. When possible,

   the salon should be located near other active _____.

3. List four location considerations when opening a salon.

   1. _____   2. _____

   3. _____   4. _____

4. Convenience of client parking should be a major consideration. If open evenings, it should be

   well _____. If in a larger city, it should be close to public _____.

5. Salons can be located near each other if each one has a different _____.

6. Before signing a lease, make sure you understand the provisions pertaining to both the

   landlord and the _____. To protect yourself, hire a _____ to help with your ne-
   gotiations.

7. What five items should a business plan include?

   1. _____

   2. _____

   3. _____

   4. _____

      _____

   5. _____

8. When you open a salon, it is important to have enough money, which is also called working

   _____.

9. Local regulations cover building _____.

10. List five items that federal laws cover:

    1. _____   2. _____

    3. _____   4. _____

    5. _____

11. Three items state laws cover are:

    1. _____   2. _____

    3. _____

12. List six items insurance covers.

    1. _____   2. _____

    3. _____   4. _____

    5. _____   6. _____

13. Identification Match: *Using the letters L P, and C (as defined below), match the correct characteristics listed below with one ownership type.*

    Key:

    I=individual ownership
    P=partnership
    C=corporation

    Characteristics:

    ___   1. ownership is shared by two or more people

    ___   2. owned by stockholders

    ___   3. proprietor receives all profits and bears all losses

    ___   4. managed by a board of directors

    ___   5. work, responsibilities, and decisions are shared

    ___   6. the state requires a charter

    ___   7. proprietor makes policies and decisions

    ___   8. each assumes each other's unlimited liability for debts

    ___   9. proprietor is owner and manager

14. Briefly list six items that should be included in an agreement when buying an established salon.

    1. _____

    2. _____

    3. _____

       _____

    4. _____

    5. _____

    6. _____

       _____

15. Simply describe three securities that should be obtained when drawing up a lease.

1. _____

2. _____

3. _____

16. List four employee information items of which you must keep accurate records.

1. _____ 2. _____

3. _____ 4. _____

17. A good business operator must always know where his/her money is being _____.

18. Of total gross income, average rent takes _____ percent, salaries and commissions take _____ percent, and the net profit is _____ percent.

19. Income is classified as receipts from services and _____ sales.

20. List seven salon expenses.

1. _____ 2. _____

3. _____ 4. _____

5. _____ 6. _____

7. _____

21. List four items that you should retain in order to keep accurate records.

1. _____ 2. _____

3. _____ 4. _____

22. Explain four reasons why business transactions must be recorded.

1. _____

2. _____

3. _____

4. _____

_____

23. List four types of records.

1. _____ 2. _____

3. _____ 4. _____

24. Supplies to be used in the daily business operations are called _____ supplies.

Those to be sold to clients are _____ supplies.

25. What should be included on a service record?

1. _____ 2. _____

3. _____ 4. _____

5. _____ 6. _____

7. _____

26. Briefly list eleven considerations for a salon's layout.

1. _____

2. _____

3. _____

4. _____

5. _____

6. _____

7. _____

8. _____

9. _____

10. _____

11. _____

OPERATING A SALON

27. The size of the salon will determine the size of the _____.

28. Cost of services is established by both the salon's location and type of _____.

29. The first thing a client sees in a salon is the _____ area.

30. The first person a client sees is the _____.

31. Scheduling appointments must make the most efficient use of time. Clients should not have

    to wait for a _____, and cosmetologists should not have to _____ for their next
    client.

32. List seven purposes of a salon telephone.

1. _____

2. _____

3. _____

4. _____

5. _____

6. _____

7. _____

33. The person making phone calls should:

    1. have a _____ voice, speak clearly, and use _____ grammar.

    2. show interest and _____

    3. be polite, respectful, and _____

    4. not say anything to irritate the _____

34. The lifeline of a salon are _____ phone calls.

35. When answering the phone:

    1. Take callers in the order that they _____.

    2. Do not talk with someone standing nearby while _____ with someone on the phone.

36. When booking appointments by phone:

    1. be familiar with all salon _____, products, and costs.

    2. be fair when making _____.

37. List three items you should use when handling complaints by phone.

    1. _____   2. _____

    3. _____

SELLING IN THE SALON

38. The first step in selling is to sell _____.

39. The foundation for suggestive selling is the manner in which you _____ each client.

40. Briefly list nine principles of selling.

    1. _____

    2. _____

    3. _____

    4. _____

    5. _____

    6. _____

    7. _____

    8. _____

    9. _____

41. Matching: *Match the client types on the left with the correct descriptions on the right.*

___ 1. shy, timid	A.	be extra courteous
___ 2. talkative	B.	start and finish quickly
___ 3. nervous, irritable	C.	explain nothing to them
___ 4. inquisitive, over-cautious	D.	don't argue with them
___ 5. know-it-all	E.	be a good listener
___ 6. teenager	F.	usually interested in current fashions
___ 7. mature	G.	take a lot of time with them
	H.	lead the conversation
	I.	argue with them
	J.	explain everything in detail

42. List three reasons why people buy services and products.

   1. _____   2. _____

   3. _____

43. When helping clients to make a decision, give them advice that is both honest and _____.

44. The best interests of the client should be your first _____.

WORD REVIEW

business plan	income tax laws	reception area
capital	individual ownership	receptionist
charter	insurance	record keeping
client types	layout	retail supplies
clientele	lease	service records
competition	local regulations	state laws
consumption supplies	location	stockholders
corporation	parking	visible
demographics	partnership	written agreements
federal laws	personnel	

FINAL REVIEW EXAMINATIONS

MULTIPLE CHOICE OR SELECTION

TEST I: MULTIPLE CHOICE OR SELECTION TEST

DIRECTIONS: Carefully read each statement. Write the letter representing the word or phrase that correctly completes the statement on the blank line to the right of the statement.

1. The practice that deals with the prevention of disease of the individual is:
    a) good grooming c) personal hygiene
    b) self-preservation d) personal development ____

2. Body odors can be prevented by regular bathing and the use of:
    a) styptics c) vapors
    b) astringents d) deodorants ____

3. To work efficiently and with a minimum of physical strain, the cosmetologist should:
    a) maintain an erect posture c) rest on client's shoulder
    b) relax by leaning on a chair d) take frequent rest periods ____

4. A wet sanitizer should contain:
    a) disinfectant solution c) antiseptic solution
    b) 30% alcohol d) 2% formalin ____

5. The most common method of sanitization in beauty salons involves:
    a) boiling water c) chemical disinfectants
    b) baking in ovens d) steam pressure sanitizers ____

6. The psychology of getting along with others is called:
    a) physical presentation c) good posture
    b) human relations d) public hygiene ____

7. Creams are removed from jars with:
    a) the end of a used towel c) a clean spatula
    b) tips of fingers d) used orangewood stick ____

8. Personal hygiene includes all of the following except:
    a) brushing your teeth c) cleansing your nails
    b) bathing or showering d) wearing the latest fashions ____

9. The first step in successful selling in the beauty salon is to:
    a) break down resistance c) sell yourself
    b) discourage competition d) be aggressive ____

10. Salon business can be effectively promoted over the telephone, provided there is:
    a) time to waste c) good planning
    b) business neglect d) sufficient capital ____

11. When calling a beauty salon, clients appreciate a receptionist who is:
    a) abrupt c) impatient
    b) indifferent d) courteous ____

12. When planning to open a beauty salon, careful consideration must be given to the selection of:
    a) a depreciation schedule
    b) students
    c) a location
    d) advertising
    ____

13. The largest expense item in operating a beauty salon is:
    a) rent
    b) salaries
    c) supplies
    d) advertising
    ____

14. A cosmetologist who repeats gossip will cause a loss of the client's:
    a) attention
    b) charm
    c) confidence
    d) posture
    ____

15. All clients must be treated honestly and fairly without showing:
    a) confidence
    b) courtesy
    c) dignity
    d) favoritism
    ____

16. The main purpose of hair and scalp treatment is to:
    a) cure canities
    b) harden the texture of hair
    c) preserve the health of the hair and scalp
    d) preserve the color of the hair
    ____

17. Thorough brushing of the scalp and hair should not be given before a:
    a) chemical service
    b) shampoo
    c) haircut
    d) scalp treatment
    ____

18. A tight scalp can be made more flexible by hair brushing and giving:
    a) an egg dry shampoo
    b) scalp manipulations
    c) a tar shampoo
    d) an antiseptic shampoo
    ____

19. In order to stimulate the scalp, massage should be given with:
    a) hacking movements
    b) vigorous manipulations
    c) gentle manipulations
    d) effleurage movements
    ____

20. Hair brushing is beneficial because it:
    a) removes dust from hair
    b) smoothes the hair cuticle
    c) stimulates blood circulation
    d) preserves hair color
    ____

21. Scalp treatments are valuable because they stimulate the:
    a) pituitary glands
    b) arrector pili
    c) blood circulation
    d) follicles
    ____

22. The skin of the body is:
    a) rigid and flexible
    b) dry and slightly rough
    c) elastic and flexible
    d) tight and inelastic
    ____

23. The skin is thinnest on the:
    a) eyebrows
    b) eyelids
    c) forehead
    d) backs of the hands
    ____

24. No blood vessels are found in the:
    a) dermis   c) subcutis
    b) cutis   d) epidermis   ____

25. The sebaceous glands secrete:
    a) melanin   c) sebum
    b) saliva   d) perspiration   ____

26. Hair is chiefly composed of a horny substance called:
    a) hemoglobin   c) keratin
    b) melanin   d) calcium   ____

27. The hair takes its shape, size, and direction from its:
    a) cortex   c) medulla
    b) cuticle   d) follicle   ____

28. The hair shaft is that portion of the hair which:
    a) projects into the skin   c) fits into the follicle
    b) projects beyond the skin   d) fits into the papilla   ____

29. The average rate of hair growth on the head is about:
    a) 1/4 inch a month   c) 1/4 inch a week
    b) 1/2 inch a month   d) 1/2 inch a week   ____

30. The appearance of a healthy nail shows a:
    a) purple color   c) yellowish color
    b) slight pink color   d) bluish color   ____

31. The part of the nail that extends over the fingertip is the:
    a) free edge   c) nail root
    b) matrix   d) nail bed   ____

32. Before applying shampoo, wet the hair with:
    a) cold water   c) warm water
    b) hot water   d) ice water   ____

33. A scalp massage during the shampoo is given with the:
    a) cushions of the fingertips c) rubber gloves
    b) metacarpus   d) ear pads   ____

34. Before draping, clients should:
    a) wash their hands   c) brush through their own hair
    b) remove their jewelry   d) remove their shoes and stockings   ____

35. Draping for a comb-out should include:
    a) a towel at the neck   c) two towels around the neck
    b) use of a shampoo cape   d) a neck strip under the cape   ____

36. The term pH stands for:
    a) potential hydrogen
    b) parts of hydroxide
    c) a natural balance
    d) phosphorus and hydrogen
    ____

37. An aniline derivative hair tint is an example of a:
    a) compound dye
    b) vegetable hair tint
    c) penetrating hair tint
    d) metallic hair dye
    ____

38. When an aniline derivative tint is mixed with hydrogen peroxide, it causes a

    chemical reaction known as:
    a) pre-softening
    b) pre-lightening
    c) oxidation
    d) neutralization
    ____

39. What type of shampoo is used on a client whose health does not permit them to

    receive a wet shampoo?
    a) medicated
    b) conditioning
    c) dry
    d) highlighting
    ____

40. To avoid overlapping in a tint retouch, color the new growth of hair about:
    a) 1/16 of an inch over the tinted hair
    b) 1/16 of an inch up to the tinted hair
    c) 1/4 of an inch over the tinted hair
    d) 1/2 of an inch up to the tinted hair
    ____

41. Temporary color rinses contain:
    a) hydrogen peroxide
    b) henna
    c) compound dyes
    d) certified colors
    ____

42. What does negative galvanic current used during a facial do to the skin?
    a) closes the pores
    b) dries the skin
    c) opens the pores
    d) removes comedones
    ____

43. Aniline derivative tints:
    a) penetrate into the hair shaft
    b) harden the hair shaft
    c) coat the hair shaft
    d) highlight the hair shaft
    ____

44. Color fillers are recommended for:
    a) virgin hair
    b) hairpieces
    c) damaged hair
    d) oily hair
    ____

45. Hair bleach does one of the following to the hair:
    a) diffuses hair pigment in the cortex
    b) adds artificial color to hair
    c) coats the hair shaft
    d) covers the natural hair pigment
    ____

46. The action of a lightener continues as long as it is:
    a) kept moist on the hair
    b) kept dry on the hair
    c) neutralized on the hair
    d) compounded on the hair   ____

47. Natural hair color is created by the reflection or _____ of light rays by melanin.
    a) absorption
    b) disintegration
    c) segregation
    d) reduction   ____

48. The sanitized end of a comedone extractor is used to remove:
    a) blackheads
    b) moles
    c) freckles
    d) birthmarks   ____

49. A facial pack is recommended for:
    a) flabby skin
    b) adding color to pale skin
    c) oily skin
    d) dry skin   ____

50. Dry skin may be caused by under-active:
    a) sudoriferous glands
    b) thyroid glands
    c) sebaceous glands
    d) salivary glands   ____

51. Before a permanent wave, a mild shampoo should be accompanied by:
    a) gentle scalp manipulations
    b) kneading scalp manipulations
    c) vibratory scalp manipulations
    d) stimulating scalp manipulations   ____

52. In selecting the cold wave solution to be used, determine the:
    a) hairststyle desired
    b) condition of the hair
    c) length of the hair
    d) color of the hair   ____

53. In cold waving, a longer processing time is usually required for hair that is:
    a) lightened
    b) tinted
    c) porous
    d) wiry   ____

54. If the fastening band is twisted or stretched too tightly in a permanent wave, it may cause a:
    a) frizzy curl
    b) springy curl
    c) hair breakage
    d) resilient curl   ____

55. End papers used in wrapping hair ends for a permanent wave must always be:
    a) non-porous
    b) waterproof
    c) porous
    d) neutralized   ____

56. The cold wave solution on the hair has a:
    a) hardening action
    b) softening action
    c) lubricating action
    d) stiffening action   ____

57. A shorter processing time in cold waving is usually required for hair that is:
   a) lightened   c) wiry
   b) resistant   d) coarse   ____

58. In giving a cold wave to tinted hair, you can expect some hair to:
   a) turn blue   c) become darker
   b) discolor   d) become longer   ____

59. In cold waving, hair that is too curly when wet and straight when dry is indicative of having been overstretched and:
   a) under-processed   c) that too much water was used
   b) over-processed   d) that too much oil was used   ____

60. A cold wave processing solution contains:
   a) quaternary ammonium   c) ammonium thioglycolate
      compound
   b) denatured ammonium   d) borax ammonium   ____

61. Which bonds in the hair must be broken down to allow the perming process to occur?
   a) disulfide   c) sulfur
   b) hydrogen   d) cortex   ____

62. The action of the chemical hair relaxer is to cause the hair to:
   a) soften and swell   c) harden and set
   b) form new curls   d) shrink   ____

63. A factor that affects the processing time of the chemical relaxer is the:
   a) stabilizer   c) hair color
   b) hair length   d) hair porosity   ____

64. The test that determines the hair's degree of elasticity is known as the _____ test.
   a) finger   c) pull
   b) match   d) relaxer   ____

65. Combing out tangles from the hair after a chemical relaxing treatment may cause hair:
   a) reversion   c) discoloration
   b) breakage   d) porosity   ____

66. The action of the chemical relaxer on the hair shaft is stopped with the application of:
   a) cream rinse   c) stabilizer
   b) cream shampoo   d) sodium hydroxide   ____

67. The two most commonly used methods of chemical hair relaxing are the thio method and the
   a) thermal method   c) single-process method
   b) sodium hydroxide method   d) gentian violet method   ____

68. Before a chemical relaxing treatment is given to a client, he/she should receive a:

    a) strand test   c) stabilizing test

    b) filler test   d) patch test   ____

69. Hair porosity is referred to as the ability of the hair to:

    a) repel moisture   c) stretch

    b) resist service   d) absorb moisture   ____

70. The best type of shampoo to use after the chemical relaxer is a/an:

    a) organic shampoo   c) toning shampoo

    b) cream shampoo   d) color shampoo   ____

71. A manicure that is not given in the manicuring area, and is often given while the client is receiving another service is called a/an _____ manicure.

    a) booth   c) plain

    b) hot oil   d) artificial   ____

72. The process of straightening over-curly hair by the use of chemical agents is known as chemical hair:

    a) neutralizing   c) relaxing

    b) stabilizing   d) stranding   ____

73. Emery boards are used to shape the:

    a) sides of the nail   c) free edge of the nail

    b) lunula   d) cuticles   ____

74. While giving a manicure, instruments should be kept in a/an:

    a) manicure table drawer   c) finger bowl

    b) alcohol jar sanitizer   d) manicurist's pocket   ____

75. To help prevent dry skin around the nails, apply:

    a) cuticle cream   c) alcohol

    b) nail polish remover d) an antiseptic   ____

76. The hair must be damp if hair shaping is done with:

    a) shears   c) a razor

    b) clippers   d) thinning scissors   ____

77. Shortening the hair in a graduated effect is known as:

    a) clipping   c) tapering

    b) singeing   d) back-combing   ____

78. Cutting the hair in graduated lengths from the nape of the neck toward the crown of the head is known as:

    a) layer cutting   c) club cutting

    b) razor cutting   d) shingling   ____

79. What type of nail polish remover should be used on plastic artificial nails?

    a) alcohol   c) acetone

    b) non-alcohol   d) non-acetone   ____

80. To offset a long neck in hair shaping it is advisable to:

    a) leave the neck exposed   c) leave the hair full at the neck

    b) give a shingle cut   d) taper the neckline short   ____

81. When holding the scissor during the haircut, which finger should be placed into the ring of the still blade?

    a) index   c) ring or third

    b) middle or center   d) thumb   ____

82. Before cutting overly curly hair, it should be shampooed, dried, and:

    a) cut with thinning shears   c) cut with a razor

    b) setting lotion should   d) an emollient product
       be applied to the hair   should be applied to the scalp and hair   ____

83. The hair that should be thinned furthest from the scalp is:

    a) fine hair   c) coarse hair

    b) medium hair   d) tinted hair   ____

84. Effilating is another term for:

    a) slithering   c) shingling

    b) clipping   d) club cutting   ____

85. The purpose of sectioning when giving a hair shaping is to:

    a) consume time   c) confuse students

    b) simplify the work   d) impress clients   ____

86. A very important objective of finger waving is to mold the hair into:

    a) high fashion coiffures   c) new hair fashions

    b) uniform ridges and waves   d) tight waves   ____

87. To develop a hairstyle that is most suitable to the client, the cosmetologist must consider:

    a) the condition of   c) waving the hair
       the client's scalp   without pin curls

    b) eliminating the necessity d) the client's features
       of waving lotion   and personality   ____

88. The stationary or immovable part of the curl, attached to the scalp, is the:

    a) stem   c) circle

    b) base   d) mobility   ____

89. When a hairstyle requires some movement, use the:

    a) on-base curl   c) no-stem curl

    b) half-stem curl   d) round-stem curl   ____

90. When hair rollers are being used, the most typical base will be:
    a) square
    c) round
    b) triangular
    d) rectangular ____

91. The size of a pin curl will determine a wave's:
    a) width
    c) direction
    b) depth
    d) ridges ____

92. A curl that decreases in size toward the hair ends is called a/an _____ curl.
    a) open center
    c) spiral
    b) forward
    d) closed center ____

93. The temperature of the pressing comb should be adjusted to the:
    a) cleanliness of the hair
    c) texture of the hair
    b) shortness of the hair
    d) length of the hair ____

94. A roller that has one end smaller than the other is known as a _____ roller.
    a) tapered
    c) mesh
    b) cylinder
    d) concave ____

95. When giving a hair pressing treatment, the cosmetologist should avoid:
    a) excessive heat and pressure
    c) pressing oil
    b) thoroughly drying the hair
    d) uniform sectioning of the hair ____

96. Frequent thermal waving may cause the hair to become:
    a) dry and lifeless
    c) oily
    b) healthier
    d) fuller ____

97. Hair burnt in thermal waving:
    a) may be reconditioned with naphtha soap
    c) may be reconditioned with peroxide
    b) may be reconditioned
    d) cannot be reconditioned with color rinse ____

98. Skills such as listening, manner of speaking, and your voice are all part of:
    a) physical presentation
    c) communication
    b) human relations
    d) professional attitude ____

99. In anchoring pin curls, all of the following are true except:
    a) clips are inserted from the open end of the shaping
    c) it is important not to disturb the shaping
    b) clips are inserted from the closed end of the shaping
    d) cotton should be placed between the skin and the clip while drying ____

100. Dryness or brittleness of wigs is prevented by:
    a) permanent waving
    c) reconditioning
    b) dry-cleaning
    d) dry shampooing ____

TEST II: MULTIPLE CHOICE OR SELECTION TEST

DIRECTIONS: Carefully read each statement. Write the letter representing the word or phrase that correctly completes the statement on the blank line to the right of the statement.

1. The cosmetologist should not discuss with the client religion or:

   a) clothes   c) politics

   b) styles   d) weather   ____

2. Clients will respect and be loyal to a cosmetologist who is:

   a) arrogant   c) sullen

   b) illiterate   d) dependable   ____

3. A good location for a beauty salon is near a:

   a) supermarket   c) bowling alley

   b) machine shop   d) tavern   ____

4. Building requirements and renovations are covered by _____ laws.

   a) local   c) income tax

   b) state   d) federal   ____

5. Good salon telephone technique requires that the receptionist should at all times be:

   a) defensive   c) apologetic

   b) tactful   d) abrupt   ____

6. When adjusting client complaints over the phone, it is important to use self-control, courtesy, and:

   a) arrogance   c) interruptions

   b) diplomacy   d) impatience   ____

7. Before people will buy beauty services or merchandise, they must be properly:

   a) endowed   c) pressured

   b) motivated   d) deceived   ____

8. Rules involving professional ethics for cosmetology include all the following except:

   a) respecting other's beliefs   c) treating everyone honestly
      and rights   and fairly

   b) being loyal to your   d) getting adequate rest
      employer/manager   and nutrition
      and coworkers   ____

9. A healthy skin should be:

   a) perfectly dry   c) slightly moist and soft

   b) without any color   d) bluish in color   ____

10. The skin is thickest on the:

    a) palms   c) forehead

    b) cheeks   d) chin   ____

11. Blood vessels, nerves, sweat and oil glands of the skin are found in the:

    a) epidermis   c) cuticle layer

    b) dermis   d) scarf layer   ____

12. The function of the sebum is to keep the skin:

    a) clean   c) dry

    b) lubricated   d) hard   ____

13. Public hygiene is also known as:

    a) personal hygiene   c) sanitation

    b) sterilization   d) disinfection   ____

14. Bad or offensive breath may be treated and minimized by:

    a) gargling with astringent   c) spraying with disinfectant

    b) spraying with a perfumed   d) gargling with an antiseptic
        caustic   ____

15. The most important consideration in personal hygiene is:

    a) personal emotion   c) ethical conduct

    b) efficiency   d) cleanliness   ____

16. Sharp metallic instruments may be sanitized with:

    a) 30% alcohol   c) 70% alcohol

    b) 50% alcohol   d) 40% alcohol   ____

17. An ultrasonic cleaner is most effective when it contains a/an:

    a) disinfectant   c) styptic

    b) active fumigant   d) deodorant   ____

18. Smelling strong chemicals:

    a) should be done before   c) may weaken their chemical
        using them   composition and strength

    b) is better than labeling   d) may irritate the membranes
        them   of the nose   ____

19. A safe antiseptic for the skin is:

    a) weaker than a disinfectant   c) carbolic acid

    b) hydrochloric acid   d) bichloride of mercury   ____

20. Scalp massage is beneficial because it stimulates the:

    a) salivary glands   c) pituitary gland

    b) blood circulation   d) thyroid gland   ____

21. An abnormal development of hair on areas of the body that normally bear only downy hair, is called all of the following except:

    a) hypertrichosis   c) lanugo

    b) superfluous   d) hirsuties   ____

22. The hair can often be reconditioned with mild shampoos, special reconditioning products, hair brushing, and:

    a) ultraviolet treatments

    b) electrolysis treatments

    c) scalp massage

    d) gentian violet jelly

    ____

23. Scalp treatments are beneficial to clients because they promote:

    a) canities

    b) a healthy scalp

    c) an increase in the hair's porosity

    d) pityriasis steatoides

    ____

24. Dry and damaged hair can be greatly improved by:

    a) emulsifying

    b) conditioning

    c) shampooing

    d) shaving

    ____

25. The primary purpose of a scalp treatment is to preserve the health of the:

    a) hair and scalp

    b) color and texture

    c) shaft and medulla

    d) cortex and cuticle

    ____

26. The first cream to be used in a plain facial is:

    a) emollient cream

    b) foundation cream

    c) cleansing cream

    d) bleaching cream

    ____

27. No face powder or cheek color should be applied after giving a/an:

    a) facial for oily skin

    b) facial for dry skin

    c) facial for normal skin

    d) acne treatment

    ____

28. The circulation of the blood is increased by applying:

    a) cleansing cream

    b) cosmetic bases

    c) facial massage

    d) good astringents

    ____

29. The main purpose of a shampoo is to:

    a) style hair easier

    b) cleanse the hair and scalp

    c) treat alopecia areata

    d) soften the scalp

    ____

30. A shampoo that has a pH of 5.5 is considered to be a/an:

    a) neutral product

    b) acid

    c) alkaline

    d) harsh shampoo

    ____

31. Clients should be referred to a physician if they have:

    a) canities

    b) an infectious disease

    c) monilethrix

    d) a noninfectious disease

    ____

32. What coats the hair to make it slick and smooth?

    a) cream rinse

    b) medicated shampoo

    c) acid rinse

    d) wig shampoo

    ____

33. A bluing rinse is used to:
    a) neutralize any yellow cast on the hair
    b) lighten the color of hair
    c) give a bluish tinge to dark hair
    d) add permanent color to the hair ____

34. An aniline derivative hair tint should not be used if there is/are:
    a) 25% gray hair
    b) abrasions of the scalp
    c) dandruff in the hair
    d) 50% gray hair ____

35. The areas usually chosen for a skin test are either behind the ear or at the inner fold of the:
    a) ankle
    b) elbow
    c) wrist
    d) neck ____

36. The action of the lightener in hair tinting continues on the hair as long as it is:
    a) rinsed out of the hair
    b) kept dry on the hair
    c) kept moist on the hair
    d) neutralized ____

37. A single application tint is prepared by mixing the required tint with:
    a) hard water
    b) 20 volume peroxide
    c) ammonia water
    d) certified color ____

38. Hair is unfit for permanent waving if it has been tinted with a/an:
    a) vegetable tint
    b) aniline derivative tint
    c) metallic dye
    d) penetrating tint ____

39. A temporary rinse lasts:
    a) five weeks
    b) four weeks
    c) until shampooed out
    d) until stripped out ____

40. Tinting lightened hair to its natural shade is known as:
    a) prelightening
    b) stripping
    c) soap cap
    d) tint back ____

41. In order to make hair porosity uniform for hair tinting, first use a:
    a) cream rinse
    b) color filler
    c) color blender
    d) color shampoo ____

42. The excessive use of hydrogen peroxide tends to make the hair:
    a) oily
    b) moist
    c) non-porous
    d) dry and brittle ____

43. A lightener retouch is applied to the:
    a) entire hair shaft
    b) hair ends
    c) new growth of hair
    d) virgin head of hair ____

44. The developing time of a hair lightener varies with the hair texture, porosity, and:
    a) time of the day
    b) altitude
    c) season of the year
    d) shade desired ____

45. No sense of feeling is found in the:

   a) skin   c) fingers

   b) hair   d) lips   ____

46. A cross-sectional view of straight hair usually reveals a/an:

   a) round shape   c) oval shape

   b) flat shape   d) square shape   ____

47. The hair root is that portion of the hair contained within the:

   a) hair cuticle   c) sweat pore

   b) hair follicle   d) hair cortex   ____

48. Coloring matter is found in the hair:

   a) medulla   c) cortex

   b) cuticle   d) follicle   ____

49. The nail plate extends from the nail root to the:

   a) lunula   c) nail bed

   b) nail matrix   d) free edge   ____

50. Nerves and blood vessels are found in the nail:

   a) plate   c) free edge

   b) bed   d) keratin   ____

51. Before applying the chemical hair relaxer, the hair must be analyzed to determine its:

   a) color, length, and direction   c) porosity, texture, and elasticity

   b) density, flow, and age   d) growth, shade, and density   ____

52. To pre-determine the results to be expected from a chemical hair relaxing treatment, it may be necessary to take a _____ test.

   a) patch   c) filler

   b) stabilizing   d) strand   ____

53. After the hair has been treated with a sodium hydroxide relaxer, and before the shampoo, the hair should be thoroughly:

   a) brushed   c) combed

   b) rinsed   d) dried   ____

54. Special perming prewrapping lotions are designed to:

   a) equalize the hair's porosity   c) be used on clients with canities

   b) add color to the hair   d) close the cuticle layer   ____

55. The main active ingredient in acid-balanced waving lotions is:

   a) ammonium thioglycolate   c) sodium hydroxide

   b) glyceryl monothioglycolate   d) hydrogen peroxide   ____

56. When analyzing hair condition, it is necessary to evaluate the hair porosity, texture, and:

   a) style   c) temperature

   b) shade   d) elasticity   ____

57. Products, such as shampoo, that are sold to clients are a/an _____ type of salon product.

   a) wholesale   c) consumption

   b) retail   d) equipment   ____

58. Hair elasticity is referred to as the ability of the hair to:

   a) repel moisture   c) absorb moisture

   b) stretch and spring back   d) resist pressure   ____

59. To stop the action and to remove as much as possible of the sodium hydroxide, the cosmetologist must give the hair a thorough:

   a) toning   c) sanitizing

   b) relaxing   d) rinsing   ____

60. Another name for the sanitizing agent sodium hypochlorite is:

   a) quats   c) bleach

   b) iodine   d) alcohol   ____

61. The stabilizer also is known as neutralizer and:

   a) thio   c) ammonium

   b) caustic   d) fixative   ____

62. Before using manicure implements, they should be:

   a) wiped with a tissue   c) cleansed and sanitized

   b) wiped with a towel   d) dipped in warm water   ____

63. 99% isopropyl alcohol is the same strength as _____ ethyl alcohol.

   a) 35%   c) 70%

   b) 60%   d) 99%   ____

64. When shaping a fingernail, the nail is filed from:

   a) corner to center   c) center to corner

   b) straight across   d) corner to corner   ____

65. Before starting a permanent wave, the hair is usually shampooed and:

   a) lubricated   c) towel dried

   b) brushed   d) lightened   ____

66. The pH of hair is:

   a) 2.5–3.5   c) 4.5–5.5

   b) 3.5–4.5   d) 7.0–8.5   ____

67. The hair sub-sections for a permanent wave should:

    a) have rectangular shapes
    c) vary all over the head
    b) have square shapes
    d) vary at the crown of the head   ____

68. If a product has a pH of 2.0, it is a/an:

    a) neutral
    c) acid
    b) balanced item
    d) alkaline   ____

69. The cold wave solution to be used is determined by the hair's:

    a) color
    c) pigment
    b) melanin content
    d) texture and porosity   ____

70. A person who has naturally light colored hair has _____ in their hair:

    a) great amounts of large
       melanin molecules
    c) an abundance of dark
       melanin molecules
    b) only large melanin
       molecules
    d) less amounts of small
       melanin molecules   ____

71. Hair that readily absorbs a cold waving solution is best described as being:

    a) porous
    c) resistant
    b) glassy
    d) wiry   ____

72. Success in permanent waving is partly due to:

    a) tight winding of the hair
    c) complete saturation of the hair
    b) under-processing of the hair
    d) over-processing of the hair   ____

73. If a permanent wave lotion accidentally drips on the skin, the cosmetologist should apply:

    a) aniline tint to the skin
    c) neutralizer to the skin
    b) formalin to the skin
    d) more lotion to the skin   ____

74. If two people each own 50% of one salon, their type of ownership is a/an:

    a) individual
    c) corporate
    b) chain salon
    d) partnership   ____

75. The most important step before giving a permanent wave is:

    a) proper hair lightening
    c) proper processing
    b) a complete color rinse
    d) hair and scalp analysis   ____

76. Human hair wigs may be properly cleansed by:

    a) dry-cleaning
    c) alkaline soap
    b) shampoo tint
    d) sodium hydroxide   ____

77. An automatic response to a stimulus is called a:

    a) mental nerve
    c) radial nerve
    b) reflex
    d) repetition   ____

78. To ensure a long lasting finger wave, mold the hair in the direction of the:

    a) hair parting

    b) hair tuft

    c) natural growth

    d) second ridge ____

79. To ensure long lasting and springy curls, the hair strand must be ribboned, stretched, and wound uniformly, and each curl:

    a) directed toward the face

    b) placed correctly on base

    c) directed away from the face

    d) placed on base in haphazard manner ____

80. That part of a pin curl found between the base and the first arc of the circle is known as the:

    a) circle

    b) stem

    c) pivot

    d) strand ____

81. To avoid splits or breaks occurring at the front or facial hairline, use:

    a) triangular bases

    b) square bases

    c) circular bases

    d) round bases ____

82. When a volume roller curl is formed, place it securely over the:

    a) stem

    b) pivot

    c) parting

    d) base ____

83. Hair lightening involves the:

    a) diffusing of natural pigment from the hair

    b) adding artificial pigment to the natural hair color

    c) restoring gray hair to its original color

    d) adding artificial pigment to pre-lightened hair ____

84. In blow waving, better waves and curls are produced with hair that has a:

    a) skip wave

    b) natural wave

    c) roller curl

    d) thermal wave ____

85. A chronic inflammatory congestion of the cheeks and nose characterized by redness and dilation of the blood vessels is called:

    a) milia

    b) asteatosis

    c) seborrhea

    d) rosacea ____

86. The technical name for fever blisters, which commonly appear on the lips, is:

    a) eczema

    b) herpes simplex

    c) rosacea

    d) pityriasis simplex ____

87. Salon and individual licenses are covered by _____ laws.

    a) federal

    b) income tax

    c) local

    d) state ____

88. The ability of a substance to resist scratching refers to its:

    a) color

    b) hardness

    c) acidity

    d) specific gravity ____

89. Proper thinning of the hair emphasizes the shape of the head and achieves the:
    a) thickness of the hair
    b) desired hairstyle
    c) length of the hair
    d) texture of the hair
    ____

90. The type of hair that can be thinned closest to the scalp is:
    a) fine hair
    b) medium hair
    c) coarse hair
    d) damaged hair
    ____

91. Lighting a match or burning wood is an example of:
    a) slow oxidation
    b) neutralization
    c) retardation
    d) rapid oxidation
    ____

92. Shears may be sanitized with:
    a) 20 volume peroxide
    b) quats
    c) sudsing
    d) carbolic acid
    ____

93. Sectioning the hair before cutting will help to achieve a/an:
    a) single hair shaping
    b) stair-step hair shaping
    c) uniform hair shaping
    d) uneven hair shaping
    ____

94. The method of cutting hair straight across without tapering is referred to as:
    a) slithering
    b) feather edging
    c) razor cutting
    d) blunt cutting
    ____

95. A fish-hooked hair end is caused when the:
    a) irons are too hot
    b) extreme ends of the hair are not caught in the irons
    c) curl is started too high
    d) curl is started too low
    ____

96. A mistake in thermal waving can be corrected by:
    a) repeated pressings until the hair is straight
    b) giving a croquignole heat curl
    c) rinsing the entire head
    d) dampening the hair and starting all over again
    ____

97. If a product has a pH of 9.5, it is a/an:
    a) neutral
    b) balanced item
    c) acid
    d) alkaline
    ____

98. A lease is an agreement between the salon owner and the:
    a) city
    b) building owner
    c) state
    d) salon employees
    ____

99. Hair brushes and combs should be cleaned and sanitized:
    a) once a day
    b) after each use
    c) whenever you have time
    d) occasionally
    ____

100. To control the hair ends when winding the hair on rollers, you may use:

a) hair spray

b) end papers

c) roller pins

d) hair clips

_____

TEST III: MULTIPLE CHOICE OR SELECTION TEST

DIRECTIONS: Carefully read each statement. Write the letter representing the word or phrase that correctly completes the statement on the blank line to the right of the statement.

1. Scalp massage should be given in the following manner:

   a) fast and without pressure

   b) slowly and without pressure

   c) slowly and with firm, steady pressure

   d) fast and with heavy pressure

   ____

2. When damaged hair and a dry tight scalp exist, the cosmetologist should recommend:

   a) a dry powder shampoo

   b) a dry liquid shampoo

   c) restyling of the hair

   d) corrective treatments

   ____

3. Most of the dust and dirt found in hair should be removed by:

   a) frequent henna applications

   b) aniline tint

   c) hair brushing

   d) vigorous shaking

   ____

4. A scalp treatment should not be given before a:

   a) shampoo

   b) permanent wave

   c) hair setting

   d) dandruff treatment

   ____

5. Another name for the sanitizing agent sodium hypochlorite is:

   a) quats

   b) iodine

   c) bleach

   d) alcohol

   ____

6. One important benefit of a scalp treatment is that it:

   a) irrigates the scalp

   b) breaks hair ends

   c) removes sebum

   d) stimulates the flow of blood

   ____

7. The cosmetologist's most important personal asset is his/her:

   a) evening clothes

   b) personality

   c) sport clothes

   d) very few friends

   ____

8. Each beauty service requires its own:

   a) room

   b) sales technique

   c) specialist

   d) salon

   ____

9. A salon owner should be protected against unexpected increases in rent by negotiating a/an:

   a) insurance policy

   b) mortgage

   c) compensation certificate

   d) lease

   ____

10. Depending on how it is used, production time of all employees may decide the difference between:

   a) satisfied patrons

   b) cooperating employees

   c) advertising media

   d) profit or loss

   ____

11. Trust and honesty are essential ingredients of professional:

    a) confidence   c) punctuality

    b) ethics   d) hygiene   ____

12. One important ingredient of a proper professional attitude is:

    a) arrogance   c) punctuality

    b) gossiping   d) aggressiveness   ____

13. Assigning a well-trained person to handle telephone calls is:

    a) wasted talent   c) business inexperience

    b) poor management   d) good planning   ____

14. An especially difficult but important telephone duty is:

    a) adjusting complaints   c) answering personal calls

    b) making social appointments   d) discouraging patrons   ____

15. A good skin complexion shows a fine, smooth texture and a:

    a) pale color   c) dry condition

    b) healthy color   d) bluish color   ____

16. The two main divisions of the skin are the epidermis and the:

    a) lucidum layer   c) corneum layer

    b) dermis   d) melanin   ____

17. The color of the skin is due to the amount of blood and coloring pigment called:

    a) keratin   c) fat

    b) melanin   d) moisture   ____

18. What should be used when massaging and lathering the client's scalp and hair during a shampoo?

    a) the cushions of the fingers   c) the palm of the hand

    b) your fingernails   d) the thumbs only   ____

19. Quaternary ammonium compound is commonly used as a:

    a) disinfectant   c) coloring

    b) styptic   d) deodorant   ____

20. A covered receptacle containing a disinfectant solution is called a/an:

    a) dry sanitizer   c) wet sanitizer

    b) cabinet sanitizer   d) oven sanitizer   ____

21. Combs and brushes are best sanitized by immersion in:

    a) a deodorant solution   c) a disinfectant solution

    b) boric acid solution   d) thio solution   ____

22. During rinsing, one finger should be over the edge of the spray nozzle in order to:
   a) monitor the water temperature
   c) determine the water pressure
   b) control the nozzle's direction
   d) hold the nozzle in place ____

23. The face and body may be kept clean by the regular use of:
   a) deodorants
   c) disinfectants
   b) soap and water
   d) germicides ____

24. To work in a salon, it is essential that the cosmetologist be free from:
   a) rheumatics
   c) canities
   b) arthritis
   d) contagious disease ____

25. In order to help preserve your teeth in a good healthy condition, it is necessary to maintain regular:
   a) use of disinfectants
   c) use of deodorants
   b) oral exercise
   d) dental care ____

26. In hair tinting, hydrogen peroxide acts as a developer when mixed with a/an:
   a) vegetable hair tint
   c) metallic hair dye
   b) aniline derivative tint
   d) compound dye ____

27. Before applying an aniline derivative haircolor, a skin or patch test is left undisturbed for a period of:
   a) 24 hours
   c) 8 hours
   b) 12 hours
   d) 7 hours ____

28. In a retouch, the hair tint is first applied to the:
   a) hair ends
   c) new growth of hair
   b) entire hair shaft
   d) hairline hairs only ____

29. Color rinses are _____ haircolorings:
   a) permanent
   c) semi-permanent
   b) temporary
   d) penetrating ____

30. In strand testing with bleaches and tints, the presence of metallic dye is indicated by immediate hair:
   a) softening
   c) thinning
   b) discoloration
   d) stripping ____

31. Rain water or water that has been chemically treated is _____ water.
   a) soft
   c) mineral
   b) hard
   d) carbonated ____

32. Thorough brushing of the scalp and hair should not be given before a/an:
   a) chemical service
   c) haircut
   b) shampoo
   d) scalp treatment ____

33. Cleansing the hair without the use of soap and water is done using a/an:
    a) liquid dry shampoo
    b) peroxide shampoo
    c) oil shampoo
    d) plain shampoo
    ____

34. What regulates the mixing of dyes and pigment to make other colors?
    a) primary colors
    b) tertiary colors
    c) the laws of color
    d) individual states, countries, or territories
    ____

35. In a lightener retouch, hair breakage may result if the:
    a) lightening formula is weak
    b) lightener overlaps
    c) lightening time is too short
    d) hair is under-lightened
    ____

36. The addition of shampoo to the lightener mixture will:
    a) slow down its action
    b) stop the lightening action
    c) hasten the lightening action
    d) spoil the lightener
    ____

37. When is the best time to apply scalp manipulations in shampooing?
    a) before lathering
    b) after the head has been dried
    c) after the head has been lathered
    d) after rinsing
    ____

38. Brittle or dry hair should be cleansed with a/an:
    a) tint shampoo
    b) drab shampoo
    c) acid-balanced shampoo
    d) dry shampoo
    ____

39. The hair's natural pigment is called:
    a) soft keratin
    b) cysteine
    c) melanin
    d) hard keratin
    ____

40. It is never advisable to brush the hair before giving a/an:
    a) cream shampoo
    b) permanent wave
    c) hair rinse
    d) acid-balanced shampoo
    ____

41. Social Security is covered under _____ laws.
    a) local
    b) state
    c) federal
    d) income tax
    ____

42. When giving a facial, eye pads should be applied before using:
    a) massage manipulations
    b) astringent lotion
    c) foundation cream
    d) red dermal light
    ____

43. After a facial, an astringent lotion is used to:
    a) lighten the skin
    b) close the pores
    c) open the pores
    d) lubricate the skin
    ____

44. Oily skin and blackheads are the result of over-active:
    a) salivary glands
    b) thyroid glands
    c) sebaceous glands
    d) sudoriferous glands

45. The nail plate is composed of a substance called:
    a) melanin   c) keratin
    b) hemoglobin   d) corpuscles   ____

46. The portion of the skin upon which the nail body rests is the:
    a) nail groove   c) nail bed
    b) cuticle   d) free edge   ____

47. The primary purpose of the hair is to:
    a) keep the scalp dry   c) keep the scalp oily
    b) keep dandruff in place   d) protect and adorn the head   ____

48. A cross-sectional view of overly-curly hair reveals almost a:
    a) flat shape   c) wavy shape
    b) round shape   d) square shape   ____

49. The lower part of the hair bulb fits over the:
    a) root   c) papilla
    b) follicle   d) shaft   ____

50. The direction of the natural flow of hair on the scalp is known as the hair:
    a) slick   c) arch
    b) stream   d) cowlick   ____

51. Brittle nails and dry cuticles are treated with a/an:
    a) oil manicure   c) regular manicure
    b) top sealer   d) machine manicure   ____

52. Manicure implements should be sanitized:
    a) once a day   c) every week
    b) after each use   d) twice a week   ____

53. Add to the water in the finger bowl a few drops of:
    a) cuticle softener   c) cuticle oil
    b) nail bleach   d) liquid soap   ____

54. What is it called when heat is created chemically within the perm product?
    a) exothermic   c) endothermic
    b) reducing agent   d) underprocessing   ____

55. What is it called when a perm is activated by an outside heat force (such as a conventional hooded hair dryer)?
    a) acid-balanced   c) exothermic
    b) reducing agent   d) endothermic   ____

56. What type of change occurs when ice melts and becomes water?
    a) chemical   c) specific gravity
    b) physical   d) mixture   ____

57. In cold waving, a test curl serves as a guide to determine the:

    a) neutralizing time   c) processing time

    b) size of hair sections   d) amount of tension to use   ____

58. During the processing time in cold waving, hair tends to:

    a) contract   c) darken

    b) expand   d) harden   ____

59. A longer processing time in cold waving is usually required for:

    a) tinted hair   c) resistant hair

    b) porous hair   d) lightened hair   ____

60. A method of wrapping a permanent wave that is suitable for extra long hair is the:

    a) double halo method   c) dropped crown method

    b) piggyback method   d) single halo method   ____

61. Stopping the action of the permanent wave solution and fixing the curl are accomplished with:

    a) a hair tint   c) 70% alcohol

    b) an oil lightener   d) a neutralizer   ____

62. An alkaline causes the hair to:

    a) harden and shrink   c) decrease in porosity

    b) soften and swell   d) increase in density   ____

63. A very mild strength permanent waving solution should be recommended for:

    a) fine hair   c) coarse hair

    b) tinted hair   d) virgin hair   ____

64. Correct wrapping in permanent waving permits better hair:

    a) porosity   c) analysis

    b) blocking   d) saturation   ____

65. In hair relaxing, what chemical agent is required in addition to the chemical relaxer?

    a) lacquer   c) waving lotion

    b) gentian violet jelly   d) neutralizing shampoo   ____

66. Before the chemical relaxing treatment, the hair should never be:

    a) rinsed   c) brushed

    b) stabilized   d) neutralized   ____

67. Before applying a thio type chemical hair relaxer, the hair should be:

    a) comb pressed   c) stabilized

    b) vigorously brushed   d) shampooed   ____

68. After a chemical relaxing treatment, a conditioner is applied:

    a) before setting the hair on rollers

    b) after setting the hair on rollers

    c) after the hair is dried and combed

    d) before the curls are combed out

    ____

69. The stabilizer is also known as neutralizer and:

    a) thio

    b) caustic

    c) ammonium

    d) fixative

    ____

70. The client's hair and scalp should be analyzed in order to determine their:

    a) condition

    b) ratio

    c) coloration

    d) oxidation

    ____

71. A hair relaxing treatment should not be done when a consultation shows the presence of scalp:

    a) looseness

    b) abrasions

    c) tightness

    d) flexibility

    ____

72. Hair texture refers to the degree of the hair's coarseness or:

    a) fineness

    b) absorption

    c) length

    d) elasticity

    ____

73. After the hair has been treated with a sodium hydroxide relaxer and before the shampoo, the hair should be thoroughly:

    a) brushed

    b) rinsed

    c) combed

    d) dried

    ____

74. Two colors situated directly across from each other on the color wheel are known as _____ colors.

    a) quaternary

    b) tone of

    c) tertiary

    d) complementary

    ____

75. When analyzing hair condition, it is necessary to evaluate the hair porosity, texture, and:

    a) style

    b) shade

    c) density

    d) elasticity

    ____

76. In order to determine which cosmetics are most suitable for the client, she should be given a complimentary:

    a) permanent wave

    b) skin analysis

    c) patch test

    d) scalp treatment

    ____

77. After a thermal wave, the hair should be combed and styled:

    a) while it is still warm

    b) after it has cooled

    c) during the thermal process

    d) after it has been waxed

    ____

78. The functional or heated parts of thermal irons include the solid round rod and the:
    a) revolving handles   c) the shank
    b) croquignole part   d) the bowl   ____

79. The least difficult type of hair for you to give a hair press is:
    a) very wiry, curly hair   c) hair with compact cuticle cells
    b) very resistant, curly hair   d) medium curly hair   ____

80. Damaged hair contains:
    a) considerable elasticity   c) considerable oil
    b) little or no elasticity   d) a very large medulla   ____

81. Burnt hair:
    a) can be reconditioned   c) can be made oily
    b) cannot be reconditioned   d) grows more rapidly   ____

82. What percent of a salon's money income is spent on employee salaries and commissions?
    a) 25%   c) 50%
    b) 30%   d) 80%   ____

83. Thinning the hair involves:
    a) cutting it straight off   c) decreasing its bulk
    b) blunt cutting   d) trimming the ends   ____

84. The process used in tapering and thinning the hair with scissors is known as:
    a) clipping   c) layer cutting
    b) razor cutting   d) slithering   ____

85. The type of salon ownership where one person owns the salon is:
    a) partnership   c) corporation
    b) individual   d) joint   ____

86. An important factor in deciding how close to the head hair may be thinned is the hair's:
    a) elasticity   c) texture
    b) color   d) stream   ____

87. A salon that is owned by stockholders and that has a state charter is known as a/an:
    a) corporation   c) partnership
    b) individual ownership   d) joint ownership   ____

88. Hair shaping implements should be sanitized:
    a) about once a week   c) daily
    b) occasionally   d) after each use   ____

89. Hair may be thinned with scissors, thinning shears, or:
    a) the clippers   c) the shank
    b) a razor   d) the pivot   ____

90. After a hair shaping, the cut hair should be placed in a/an:
    a) waste basket
    c) corner of booth
    b) open container
    d) closed receptacle   ____

91. The two divisions of the autonomic nervous system are the sympathetic and _____ systems.
    a) parasympathetic
    c) central nervous
    b) peripheral
    d) apathetic   ____

92. If a product has a pH of 2.0, it is a/an:
    a) neutral
    c) acid
    b) balanced item
    d) alkaline   ____

93. A hairpiece with a flat base that is used in special areas of the head is a:
    a) dart
    c) wiglet
    b) switch
    d) swirl wig   ____

94. If a salon is sold, the sales agreement should contain within it all of the following except:
    a) a written purchase agreement
    c) a guarantee of profits to be made
    b) an inventory statement
    d) the owner's identity   ____

95. The three principal parts of a pin curl are the base, the circle, and the:
    a) texture
    c) stem
    b) elasticity
    d) mobility   ____

96. When the hairstyle requires a great deal of mobility, use the:
    a) full-stem curl
    c) no-stem curl
    b) half-stem curl
    d) round-stem curl   ____

97. Pin curls, placed behind the ridge-line of shaping, are called:
    a) roller curls
    c) pivot curls
    b) ridge curls
    d) sculpture curls   ____

98. To create the illusion of decreasing the width of the forehead, recommend:
    a) a center part
    c) bangs
    b) a side part
    d) short hair   ____

99. Pin curls, formed in a shaping, should be:
    a) dry
    c) overlapped
    b) elongated
    d) spaced apart   ____

100. The ideal facial shape is the:
    a) oval
    c) oblong
    b) square
    d) pear   ____

ANATOMY

DIRECTIONS: Carefully read each statement. Write the letter representing the word or phrase that correctly completes the statement on the blank line to the right of the statement.

1. The more fixed attachment of a muscle is called:
   a) origin of muscle   c) muscle tone
   b) insertion of muscle   d) ligament   ____

2. The epicranus muscle covers the:
   a) side of head   c) bottom of skull
   b) top of skull   d) cheekbone   ____

3. The nervous system controls and coordinates all body:
   a) structures   c) diseases
   b) functions   d) cleanliness   ____

4. The cerebro-spinal nervous system controls the:
   a) stomach muscles   c) involuntary muscles
   b) heart muscles   d) voluntary muscles   ____

5. The trifacial is the chief sensory nerve of the:
   a) arm   c) chest
   b) face   d) shoulder   ____

6. The temporal nerve affects the muscles of the forehead, temple, and:
   a) nose   c) lower lip
   b) upper lip   d) eyebrows   ____

7. Vessels that carry blood away from the heart are called:
   a) veins   c) capillaries
   b) arteries   d) eyebrows   ____

8. The fluid part of the blood is called:
   a) plasma   c) red blood cells
   b) white blood cells   d) thrombocytes   ____

9. The common carotid artery is located at the side of the:
   a) head   c) neck
   b) crown   d) nose   ____

10. The frontal artery supplies the:
    a) back of the head   c) forehead
    b) crown   d) side of nose   ____

11. The wrist bones are called the:
    a) carpal bones   c) digital bones
    b) metacarpal bones   d) radial bones   ____

12. The skeletal system is important because it:

    a) covers and shapes the body   c) provides bony framework to the body

    b) supplies the body with blood   d) carries nerve messages   ____

13. The occipital bone forms the back and base of the:

    a) neck   c) upper jaw

    b) cranium   d) forehead   ____

14. The flat expanded tendon connecting one muscle to another is called:

    a) involuntary muscle   c) voluntary muscle

    b) aponeurosis   d) fascia   ____

15. The muscular system is dependent for its activities upon the skeletal system and the:

    a) lymphatic system   c) nervous system

    b) digestive system   d) circulatory system   ____

16. The orbicularis oris is a muscle that closes the:

    a) eyes   c) nostrils

    b) lips   d) ears   ____

17. The sensory nerves carry messages from the:

    a) brain to muscles   c) brain to spinal cord

    b) sense organs to the brain   d) brain to the bones   ____

18. Twelve pairs of cranial nerves branch out from the brain and reach various parts of the:

    a) arms and hands   c) abdomen and back

    b) legs and feet   d) head, face, and neck   ____

19. The seventh cranial nerve is the chief motor nerve of the:

    a) arm   c) face

    b) chest   d) shoulder   ____

20. Blood cells that fight harmful bacteria are called:

    a) platelets   c) red corpuscles

    b) white corpuscles   d) thrombocytes   ____

21. The superior labial artery supplies the:

    a) chin   c) upper lip

    b) lower lip   d) back of ear   ____

22. The parietal bones form the top and sides of the:

    a) face   c) cheeks

    b) cranium   d) neck   ____

23. The frontal bone forms the:

    a) upper jaw   c) forehead

    b) lower jaw   d) cheek   ____

24. The ulnar nerve supplies the:
    a) thumb side of the arm
    b) little finger side of the arm
    c) back of the hand
    d) top side of the fingers   ____

25. The palm of the hand contains:
    a) 8 carpal bones
    b) 5 metacarpal bones
    c) 10 phalanges
    d) dorsal bones   ____

26. One of the functions of the muscular system is to:
    a) circulate the blood
    b) nourish the body
    c) produce body movements
    d) produce marrow   ____

27. One of the functions of bones is to:
    a) contract muscles
       to the body
    b) expand muscles
    c) give strength and shape
    d) stimulate blood circulation   ____

28. The temporal bones form the:
    a) forehead
    b) lower jaw
    c) Adam's apple
    d) sides of the head   ____

29. Maxillae are bones that form the:
    a) lower jaw
    b) upper jaw
    c) eye sockets
    d) forehead   ____

30. Muscles controlled by the will are called:
    a) involuntary muscles
    b) voluntary muscles
    c) cardiac muscles
    d) non-striated muscles   ____

31. The epicranus consists of two parts, the frontalis and the:
    a) corrugator
    b) caninus
    c) risorius
    d) occipitalis   ____

32. The main divisions of the nervous system are the sympathetic, peripheral, and the:
    a) lymphatic system
    b) ganglia system
    c) spinal cord
    d) cerebro-spinal system   ____

33. The skin of the lower lip and chin is supplied by the:
    a) infra-orbital nerve
    b) supra-orbital nerve
    c) mental nerve
    d) auricular nerve   ____

34. The seventh cranial nerve is also known as the:
    a) facial nerve
    b) trifacial nerve
    c) trigeminal nerve
    d) cervical nerve   ____

35. Vessels that carry blood back to the heart are called:
    a) veins
    b) capillaries
    c) arteries
    d) lacteals   ____

36. Blood cells carrying oxygen to the body are called:
    a) white corpuscles   c) red corpuscles
    b) blood platelets   d) hemoglobin   ____

37. Those parts of the body not reached by the blood are nourished by:
    a) sweat   c) juices
    b) sebum   d) lymph   ____

38. The lower region of the face is supplied by the:
    a) occipital artery   c) posterior artery
    b) facial artery   d) frontal artery   ____

39. The submental artery supplies the:
    a) chin   c) nose
    b) ear   d) upper lip   ____

40. The external jugular vein returns the blood to the heart from the:
    a) brain   c) head and face
    b) shoulders   d) chest   ____

41. The zygomatic or malar bones form the:
    a) outer walls of the nose   c) cheeks
    b) mouth   d) "U" shaped bone in throat   ____

42. The mandible bone forms the:
    a) upper jaw   c) cheek
    b) lower jaw   d) head   ____

43. The orbicularis oculi is a muscle that surrounds the margin of the:
    a) mouth   c) eye socket
    b) nose   d) head   ____

44. The mentalis is a muscle located in the:
    a) upper lip   c) jaw
    b) eyelid   d) chin   ____

45. The heart, lungs, liver, kidneys, stomach, and intestines are body _____ .
    a) systems   c) organs
    b) tissues   d) secretions   ____

46. Nerves going to all parts of the body originate in the brain and the:
    a) sense organs   c) spinal cord
    b) muscles   d) heart   ____

47. The zygomatic motor nerve affects the muscles of the upper part of the:
    a) mouth   c) chin
    b) cheek   d) nose   ____

48. The back flow of blood in the veins is prevented by:

    a) valves   c) vesicles

    b) vessels   d) vehicles   ____

49. The supra-orbital artery supplies the:

    a) lip   c) forehead

    b) nose   d) ear   ____

50. The occipital artery supplies blood to the region of the:

    a) back of head   c) front of head

    b) mouth and nose   d) cheeks   ____